Talking Men's Health

"This will be a tremendous resource for both practitioners and researchers working in the field. Research has consistently shown that in issues such as coping, mental wellbeing, and self-management support, men who live with long term conditions often have specific needs and preferences and require a tailored approach. This text will provide nurses and allied health professionals with invaluable knowledge to better understand men's needs and improve their delivery of person-centred care."

—Paul Galdas, Professor of Nursing and Men's Health, *University of York, UK*

"A very clever book that covers a breadth of important issues in relation to men's health while also providing the critical nuance and depth that is required when considering the complex issues involved in this field. A must read for anyone with a genuine interest in moving men's health forward."

—Steve Robertson, Emeritus Professor of Men, Gender and Health, *University of Sheffield, UK*

"This is a very important book in the growing field of men's health. Little has been written on the experiences of men with chronic ill-health and this text, based on interviews with men with rheumatoid arthritis and systemic sclerosis, gives a clear indication of the challenges men face with life-changing conditions. The honesty with which the men open up to describe their day-to-day realities gives an insight that all working within the health and social care sector should read and learn from."

—Alan White, Emeritus Professor of Men's Health, *Leeds Becket University, UK*

"An engaging and accessible handbook to the many intricacies of men's health. Centering the words and experiences of male patients themselves, Caroline Flurey guides us deftly through the interplay of masculinity, male identity and men's relationship to their health and their bodies. A book that demands a place on the shelves of every clinician and academic with an interest in men's health and wellbeing."

—Ally Fogg, writer and co-founder of Men & Boys Coalition

"As a health researcher, I've come to understand that beneath the resilient exteriors society expects, men deeply desire understanding and support as they navigate their health challenges. This book is a pioneering testament to their stories, the first of its kind to call for dismantling the barriers of silence and stigma. It aims to foster environments where men can openly discuss their health, revealing their vulnerabilities without fear of judgment. By spotlighting men's unique experiences with long-term conditions, we challenge damaging societal narratives and advocate for health support systems that are both inclusive and effectively tailored to their needs."

—Yeliz Prior, Professor of Clinical Rehabilitation,
University of Salford, UK

"This book explores how men experience long-term health conditions. It challenges the stereotype that men are unemotional about their health and explores the impact illness can have on masculinity, mental well-being, body image, and intimacy. As a female researcher, Caroline provides a unique and nuanced perspective on how men cope with long-term conditions, from self-management strategies to navigating the sometimes difficult decision to seek help.

Packed with practical advice, this book is an indispensable resource for healthcare professionals, researchers, and anyone committed to providing comprehensive and compassionate care for men with long-term health conditions."

—Mwidimi Ndosi, Associate Professor of Rheumatology Nursing,
University of the West of England, UK

Caroline Flurey

Talking Men's Health

Understanding and Supporting Men with Long-Term Conditions

palgrave
macmillan

Caroline Flurey
Bristol, UK

ISBN 978-3-031-62592-3 ISBN 978-3-031-62593-0 (eBook)
https://doi.org/10.1007/978-3-031-62593-0

This Palgrave Macmillan imprint is published by the registered company Springer Nature Switzerland AG.
The registered company address is: Gewerbestrasse 11, 6330 Cham, Switzerland

Paper in this product is recyclable.

For Toby, may understanding and support for men's health grow faster than you do

Acknowledgements

First, a huge thank you to the men who gave me your time and trust to share your stories. Without you this book would not have been possible, and I hope I've done your experiences justice. I'm grateful to clinical teams who facilitated access, and those who remind me of the importance of this work every time you ask how to improve care for men. Thank you to all those who have paved the way in advocating for the importance of men's health and wellbeing, and who laid an evidence-base for me to build on. I'm ever grateful to have the shoulders of such impressive giants to stand on. Thank you to my funders: Versus Arthritis, and World Scleroderma Foundation and Association des Sclerodermique de France who funded the underpinning research for this book; and University of the West of England, Bristol, for contributing time for writing. Thank you to my Palgrave editors: Grace Jackson for seeing the potential in this book to commission it, and Clelia Petracca for supporting me through to completion.

Thank you to many supportive and inspiring colleagues and students, too numerous to name individually, for listening to my ideas, bringing fresh perspectives, and challenging my imposter syndrome. Especially to Prof Nicki Walsh, Prof Fiona Cramp, Prof Emma Dures, Dr Mwidimi Ndosi, and Prof Peter Clegg for helping reignite my passion for research; and to my fellow Trustees of Men & Boys Coalition, who constantly expand my knowledge of men and boys' issues. The voices of those who have shaped my thoughts and writing as supervisors, collaborators, co-authors, and patient research partners are woven throughout these pages.

I'm eternally grateful to Prof Sarah Hewlett, Dr Maz Morris, Dr Jon Pollock, Dr Rod Hughes, Prof Alan White, Prof John Kirwan, Prof Karen Rodham, Prof Paul Galdas, Pam Richards, and Bob Noddings for your expertise and guidance throughout my career.

Thank you to wonderful friends and family for your support. I can't name you all, but you know who you are; thank you for putting up with me. Special mentions: To my four-legged ginger co-author, Rufus, always by my side when things are hardest, mostly because he likes the taste of salty tears. To Auntie Lynn for not giving up on me when I shut down, and Nathan McIntyre who has never been far from my mind while writing this. To Mark Zachary, for reading Dr Seuss to me when the world was ending. You'll be happy to hear I haven't mentioned the patriarchy once. To Dr Bethan Jones, my flamingling, for searching for imaginary birds with me and holding me accountable since the very beginning. To Prof Yeliz Prior, for being the big sister I always wanted, seeing so much more in me than I see in myself, and being a constant inspiration. Finally, I owe so much to the opportunities and support that my parents have given me. Mum, thank you for passing on your love of learning to me. I wish you could see this, you'd have been so incredibly proud. Dad, thank you for holding my hand through the darkness, and always believing in me.

Contents

CHAPTER 1

Introduction

There is a prevailing public narrative that says men are strong, stoic, and silent, and never more so than in matters relating to their health and well-being. The more this unhelpful narrative is repeated, the more we reinforce to men and boys that to talk about their health would be to deviate from how 'real' men or 'normal' men behave. This book reinforces the idea that when given permission and provided with the right environment men *will* talk about their health. Within this book I will focus on different aspects of living with long-term conditions and how men talk about their experiences with each of these. I will be drawing on examples from my own research with men with rheumatoid arthritis and systemic sclerosis and looking to the existing literature on men with long-term conditions. I will also aim to challenge unhelpful societal assumptions about men and their approach to health along the way. Whilst men are often branded as 'hard to reach' this book takes the stance men are under-served by health services. It includes implications for practice and suggestions for engaging men with long-term conditions in support for their health and mental health.

1.1 Why Does Men's Health Matter?

Men are more likely to die prematurely than women at all ages, and of all causes (White et al., 2011), including 75% of completed suicides being men (Freeman et al., 2017). This feeds into a public narrative that says

C. Flurey, *Talking Men's Health*,
https://doi.org/10.1007/978-3-031-62593-0_1

men are poor at looking after their health (Courtenay, 2000). However, as I will discuss and give examples of throughout this book, when given appropriate settings and support men can and do engage actively with their health (Galdas et al., 2014, 2015). It could be argued that in many areas of life things have been built by men for men. However, when it comes to healthcare men are often an under-served group, with social and institutional barriers in place that make it harder for men to engage with health services in a way that works for them.

We know there are gender differences when it comes to coping with illness, with men experiencing specific challenges in coping with and managing long-term health conditions (del Mar García-Calvente et al., 2012; McCaughan et al., 2011). For example, in rheumatoid arthritis, men tend to use fewer and less diverse coping strategies and self-management techniques than women, and they tend to take longer to adjust and adapt to living with the condition (Flurey et al., 2016a). However, men are rarely the focus of targeted health and self-management support interventions, and data from 34 countries in the European Union (including the UK as this was pre-Brexit) suggests that 'men need their own health strategy' (White et al., 2011). Men are likely to be better served with more tailored healthcare provision that addresses the way they prefer to engage with and receive healthcare, and that addresses issues that matter to them. With the passing of the Equality Act in 2010 (Equality Act, 2010) there is a legal requirement for care to reflect the differing needs of men and women, which has prompted closer examination of men's experiences of service provision.

When I began writing this book, the UK government were in the midst of an inquiry into men's health, and key players in the men's health and wellbeing sector have been calling for a UK men's health strategy for a number of years. On International Men's Day 2023, the UK government announced plans to appoint a men's health ambassador and have now launched a men's health task and finish group to improve men's access to and engagement with healthcare services, including increasing the uptake of NHS health checks. The shadow health secretary has also recently announced that the Labour Party is looking to include a men's health strategy in their election manifesto. Whilst there's still a long way to go, men's health has never had more attention, so it couldn't be timelier to think about men with long-term conditions.

By understanding men's experience of illness, we can begin to address how health services and support can be improved to better meet their needs. Exploring how men talk about their health is crucial to furthering our understanding of: what's important to men, what do they struggle with, how are they currently coping and managing, what do they need help with, what would that help ideally look like, and what do they want their healthcare professionals to know?

1.2 Focus of the Book

Long-term conditions (also known as chronic diseases or chronic illnesses) are ongoing conditions that there is currently no cure for, are managed with medical treatment, and affect activities of daily living. Around 15 million people in England are living with a long-term condition (Department of Health, 2012). Once diagnosed, patients often have to learn to live with and manage these for the rest of their lives. Thus, men with long-term conditions may have a different relationship with health and healthcare from those men dealing with an acute illness or injury. Additionally, strategies for engaging men with long-term conditions in support services may differ from targeting men in public health outreach such as screening programmes or preventative healthcare due to their ongoing existing relationship with healthcare. This book aims to address how men talk about their experiences with long-term conditions, how they cope and self-manage, and their support needs and preferences. Understanding this may be a positive step towards improving care and support services for men with long-term conditions.

My own primary research has been with men with rheumatic diseases, so I am using this as the starting point for this book. Thematic analysis of my interviews and focus groups with men with rheumatoid arthritis and systemic sclerosis have previously been published elsewhere (Flurey et al., 2016b, 2018b, 2022). In the current book rather than using the themes from this analysis, the chapters are structured around key elements of living with a long-term condition that men have talked about throughout my own qualitative research and the literature.

Within each chapter of this book my starting point is the findings from my own research, which I then broaden out to understand what we know from the literature from other long-term conditions. This book particularly focuses on the qualitative literature (descriptive experiences rather than numbers: primarily interviews, focus groups, and open-text responses) to ground this in what men with long-term conditions are telling us about their health.

This book focuses on men's experiences, self-management, coping, and support needs rather than the physiological impact of long-term conditions. Thus, gender is more relevant than sex to these topics of discussion. So, when I talk about men, I mean this as inclusively as possible to mean anyone who identifies as man. However, it is important to highlight that whilst some research exists on trans-men within a health context, research on trans-men in long-term conditions is almost non-existent and relates more to screening and treatment than experiences and support needs. This has resulted in this book reflecting the voices of cis men, which I acknowledge as a limitation.

There are various competing philosophical approaches to discussing men's health, so it is perhaps helpful to explain that my personal stance is a combination of social constructionism and critical realism. Social constructionism views reality as socially constructed, implying that what we perceive as real or true is shaped by social processes, language, and cultural context. In the context of men's health, societal norms and cultural expectations, such as 'men don't seek help' or 'men don't talk', can influence how men perceive and express their masculinity, which can in turn impact their health behaviours. On the other hand, critical realism emphasises the underlying social, economic, and environmental factors that contribute to the construction of masculinity and their impact on men's health outcomes. For example, critical realism recognises that men from marginalised socioeconomic backgrounds may face unique challenges and pressures related to employment, financial stability, and social status, which can shape their sense of masculinity and influence their approach to their health.

Some academics may take an evolutionary perspective, viewing masculinity as a set of traits and behaviours that have been shaped by evolutionary processes. For example, the suggestion that physical strength and aggression may have evolved as advantageous traits for competing with other males for access to mates and resources, and for defending against potential threats. However, this is not addressed throughout this book as it overlooks the role of culture, socialisation, and individual differences, which may offer a more comprehensive understanding. Additionally, acceptance of evolutionary explanations in the context of disability has the potential to contribute to negative perceptions and enhance stigma.

1.3 What Is Hegemonic Masculinity?

At times throughout this book, I'll refer to the concept of 'hegemonic masculinity'—so what is it? Hegemonic masculinity is a concept that relates to the current most honoured way of defining being a man in any particular locale. As a sociological construct, hegemonic masculinity seeks to explain how and why men maintain dominant societal roles over women, or other gendered identities perceived as feminine. Connell argues that masculinity is not a singular, fixed identity but rather a complex and diverse set of social practices that are shaped by power dynamics, cultural norms, and historical contexts. In many societies traits such as being 'tough, independent, unemotional, physically competent, mentally strong [and] aggressive' are idealised as the epitome of what it means to be a man (Connell, 2005; Connell & Messerschmidt, 2005). However, hegemonic masculinity is not just a collection of individual attributes but a shared social ideal that is reinforced and maintained through various institutions and practices. Connell's concept of hegemonic masculinity recognises that multiple 'masculinities' exist, which can vary depending on societal and cultural influences as well as individual differences.

Only a minority of men will enact hegemonic masculinity as it is more of an ideal than achievable, but the concept suggests men position themselves in relation to this. Men who benefit from and support dominant forms of masculinity without actively participating in a strong version of masculine dominance can be considered to be displaying 'complicit masculinity'. Connell suggests that 'complicit masculinity' operates through subtle mechanisms, such as conformity to traditional gender roles. Men who embody 'complicit masculinity' may not actively challenge or resist dominant forms of masculinity, even if they recognise the harm they cause or the privilege they possess. Positioned against hegemonic masculinity, Connell (Connell, 2005) describes 'marginalised masculinities' and 'subordinated masculinities'.

'Marginalised masculinities' describes men who may not conform to the idealised norms associated with hegemonic masculinity and may be devalued or marginalised as a result. This inability to benefit from dominant forms of masculinity can be due to barriers imposed by social, cultural, or individual differences such as social class, ethnicity, or abilities. However, these men may still subscribe to or enact the practices of hegemonic masculinity, such as aggression or suppression of emotions. Men living with a long-term condition could be considered as sitting within 'marginalised masculinities' as the limitations imposed by a long-term condition may force them to deviate from idealised norms of hegemonic masculinity.

'Subordinated masculinities' are distinct from 'marginalised masculinities' as these men may be seen as rejecting (some or all) traditional masculine values. These are men who display traits that are the opposite of hegemonic ideals such as physical weakness and open displays of emotions and are devalued or subordinated as a result of this. Gay men are the most commonly cited example of subordinated masculinity in the literature. In many societies, hegemonic masculinity is closely tied to heteronormative ideals. This means that for gay men who deviate from these norms, their masculinity may be treated as lesser within the broader hierarchy of dominant masculinities. They may therefore face discrimination, stigma, and marginalisation due to their sexual orientation and failure to conform to societal expectations of masculinity. There is hope for this changing over time, with some researchers suggesting there may be a decline in homophobia's ability to define masculinity as heteronormative in younger generations (McCormack & Anderson, 2010).

Now, if you're thinking 'I just about understand this, but I wish someone would explain it to me in Game of Thrones (GoT) terms' then look no further; Aurita and Huda (2018) have got you covered. In the seven kingdoms of GoT, hegemonic masculinity is typified by the knights; they set the standard for the epitome of masculinity. Men admire them, women desire them, and boys aspire to be them. This is exemplified by Jamie Lannister who is strong, competent, and hot-tempered. Despite character flaws he never sees great consequences and consistently benefits from his masculine status. Jon Snow, illegitimate son of the Lord of Winterfell, is our marginalised masculinity exemplar. In nearly every way Jon Snow enacts the hegemonic masculine ideal. Like Jamie, he is strong, competent, and brave. However, Jon is unable to benefit in the same way due to his social status as a bastard: he is denied opportunities and recognition. Finally, for subordinated masculinity we have Samwell Tarly, who openly displays emotion including fear and even publicly cries and admits to being a coward. Thus, despite being the first-born son of a Lord, his behaviours associated with feminine traits cause him to be bullied and outcast by those who value hegemonic masculine ideals. Another example is Lord Varys, a eunuch. His appearance and manner are effeminate and thus he is belittled and mocked. Varys is a powerful man due to the information he possesses about key players, but this is often overlooked due to him being regarded as feminine, abnormal, or deviant (Aurita & Huda, 2018).

The concept of hegemonic masculinity has been both widely used and widely debated, and the purpose of this book is not to debate its accuracy or usefulness in relation to men with long-term conditions. I have described it here as it provides a useful lens through which to consider the impact of long-term conditions on men. It is important to consider that when learning to live with a long-term condition, men may also be coming to terms with redefining their own masculinity or reconsidering their masculine status in a hierarchy of masculinities, within the context of newfound limitations. This may have wider implications with men with long-term conditions potentially finding themselves needing to re-assess their social standing and self-worth, which will be discussed throughout this book.

In hegemonic masculinity (society's current most honoured way of being a man), men are supposed to be strong, stoic, and silent in matters relating to their health (Courtenay, 2000). The desire to conform to hegemonic masculine ideals can make it difficult for men to participate in behaviours that deviate from these, such as talking about their health. However, as this book will demonstrate, when directly asked and given space to talk in safe environments, men will talk about their health. Moreover, men will talk openly and candidly about not just physical but also emotional impact of living with a long-term condition.

1.4 Why Am I Interested in Men's Health?

I'm often asked how (as a woman) I ended up researching men's health. Well, like all the best things in life, I fell into it. As Tim Minchen says in his '9 life lessons' address at the University of Western Australia graduation for his honorary doctorate: *"Put your head down and work with pride on whatever is in front of you. You never know where you might end up. Just be aware the next worthy pursuit will probably appear in your periphery, which is why you should be careful of long-term dreams. If you focus too far in front of you, you won't see the shiny thing out the corner of your eye"*. I didn't come to men's health through a family tragedy, or personal experience, I'd never intended to focus on this. Men were simply the shiny thing out of the corner of my eye. Or to put it another way, it was purely evidence driven.

My PhD focused on what daily life was like for patients with rheumatoid arthritis. A recent medication break-through had given us biologics, a sub-type of disease-modifying anti-rheumatic drugs that work by interfering with the autoimmune process. My PhD was interested in how patients now experienced life on these current more aggressive medications, their self-management behaviours in both daily life and when experiencing disease flares (uncontrollable, exacerbated symptoms), and the decision-making process in seeking medical help for disease flares.

One of my PhD studies used a method called Q-methodology (Watts & Stenner, 2012). Q-methodology was designed to create a systematic way of exploring the subjectivity (beliefs, feelings, and opinions) of any issue that a range of views can be held about. Q-methodology involves participants sorting statements of opinion about a particular issue according to how much they agree with those statements. We also collect comments from participants about the way they sort the statements to help understand their reasoning and add context. Participants are then correlated by the way they sort the statements to produce clusters of different opinions or ways of looking at a particular issue (called 'factors' in Q-methodology). If you're familiar with factor analysis it may help to understand Q-methodology as a reversed form of factor analysis where the participants themselves become the factors according to the way they have sorted the statements (rather than the individual statement items). Using this method in my PhD studies I asked participants to sort statements based on the literature and my interviews with patients. I found one group of participants who were struggling to cope with rheumatoid arthritis and weren't keen on the support currently on offer within rheumatology. On looking at the demographic data for the participants in each group I was surprised to find this struggling group was made up of all the men who had taken part in my study (Flurey et al., 2014a).

When it came time to decide which direction to take my research at the end of my PhD the focus on men was an obvious next step. This led to a three-year post-doctoral fellowship funded by Arthritis Research UK (now Versus Arthritis) to explore the experiences, coping strategies, and support needs of men with rheumatoid arthritis, which laid the groundwork for my subsequent work on men with systemic sclerosis and overall interest in men with long-term conditions.

1.5 Talking to Men

Most of the men who have taken part in my studies seem to have had a positive experience of talking about their health to me on their own (in interviews) or with other patients (in focus groups). This has been particularly notable for focus groups where they often comment on the benefits of being able to meet other men with the same condition as them—to share and compare their own experiences and to learn from each other. For many of the men in my focus groups this was the first opportunity they'd had to talk to another man (and for some another patient at all) with the same condition. Support is not the purpose of research, and we would never promise this as a benefit to taking part, yet many of the men did seem to get a lot out of these. For some of my focus groups men even swapped email addresses with each other at the end to continue sharing advice. When I later discuss support in Chap. 9, we'll learn that men like support to have a clear purpose. The nature of taking part in a research study provided these men with a clear purpose to attending and contributing, so it is perhaps unsurprising that a by-product of these was a form of support.

Although men who have participated tend to report a positive experience it can be difficult to encourage men to take part in health research studies. This is particularly the case for research studies that focus on psychological or social aspects of a condition and even more so for those that involve talking about themselves (qualitative methods). This means I'm often asked by other researchers for advice on how to increase their numbers of male participants. So, in this section I'll talk a little about what worked for me in encouraging men to take part, and once they'd agreed what worked in getting them talking.

First, there's the obvious issue of being a woman researching men. In Chap. 9 I'll discuss men having different preferences as to the gender of their treating healthcare professionals. This lack of consensus on gender preference is no different for talking to men for research purposes, and for this reason there's no clear answer in the literature either. Whilst men with penile cancer have expressed concerns about telling their story to a female researcher (Witty et al., 2014), men with anxiety have expressed preferences for female researchers perceiving them as more empathetic (Gough et al., 2021). It has also been suggested that a male researcher may encourage male participants to (over)emphasise masculine traits to reduce perceived power imbalances and exert control or dominance (Broom &

Cavenagh, 2010; Oliffe & Mróz, 2005; Schwalbe & Wolkomir, 2001). This positioning is also worth considering in the focus group environment as the men may be performing for each other. As Frosh observes with his interviews and focus groups with boys, none of these interactions would necessarily be more authentic than each other; they are simply different ways of men presenting themselves depending on their audience (Frosh et al., 2002). There may well be men who didn't take part in my studies as the idea of talking to a (younger) woman could have been off-putting. However, on the other hand there may have been times when I was told things they might not have felt comfortable telling a male researcher or their healthcare professionals (Richards & Emslie, 2000).

In recruiting men to take part in my studies they were initially given information or introduced to me by a member of their clinical team. This provided a form of legitimacy for the study as it came with a recommendation from their healthcare professional as a worthy piece of research. Anecdotally—in my own experiences of recruiting patients to studies—I would suggest men are more likely to take part if they can see a clear purpose and assess it as a good use of their time. This introduction from a member of the clinical team went a long way towards validating the benefits and purpose of the study. Additionally, many men who took part also expressed a positive relationship and level of support from their clinical team and wanted to give back. Thus, using gatekeepers who are valued by men for their expertise is a key first step in encouraging men's participation in research. Thinking about gatekeepers, I also found men's partners to be helpful in encouraging men to take part. They were even sometimes the ones to phone me to arrange the time and place.

Keeping in mind men like things to have a clear purpose, this needs to be apparent from the information you give them about the study. It's important to emphasise the value and potential impact of the work. My studies have all focused specifically on men, and some men have told me they've taken part for this reason ("*I wouldn't normally take part in this sort of thing, but you're looking for men so I couldn't step back and leave it to the women this time [laughs]*", Frank, rheumatoid arthritis). So even if you're looking for a mixed gender sample, I would suggest there's a lot of value in targeted recruitment to tell men you need them specifically. In recruiting young men, one of my PhD students Ruben McNeil-Walsh tried including quotes from earlier interviews in his advertising materials, which seemed to work well. This may provide validation in illustrating to potential participants that this is something other men are taking part in, as well as demystifying the topics that will be under discussion.

Once in the interviews or focus groups I started with a broad question (e.g., 'Tell me what it's like to be a man with rheumatoid arthritis'). This allowed the men to take the question in whichever direction they felt most comfortable, which often started with a description of symptoms. In focus groups this enabled men to compare symptoms and medication with each other, which helped them build rapport and confidence discussing 'safe' topics. In groups I tended to find it was worth setting aside around 30 minutes to enable men to 'bed in' with these topics, which also provided them with a benefit to taking part as they were able to learn and share with each other.

Moving on to more sensitive topics such as death or sex and intimacy, I found men were generally responsive to direct questions. They often seemed to welcome the opportunity to talk about these without having to be the ones to bring up the issues. My mum had died a few months before my systemic sclerosis focus groups, so I was used to talking quite directly about death and perhaps this helped these discussions to be so frank. I was less confident in directly asking men about sex and intimacy with worries about embarrassing them but gained confidence in this as the focus groups continued and I saw their willingness to talk, with men often raising these issues themselves. In talking about the emotional impact, men's willingness to open up was often a domino effect once one man in the group got the ball rolling. In my focus groups with men with rheumatoid arthritis some of these were co-facilitated by a patient research partner and men tended to respond well to him opening up first and then asking whether they experienced anything similar. This provided a form of permission and legitimacy that this was a safe trusted space to share. It also gave them confidence to see other men who opened up were listened to and supported.

These are some of the things that worked for me, and I'm still continually learning and trying new things. Importantly, as you'll see throughout this book, men did open up in my interviews and focus groups, and also to the authors of the studies I cite. You will also see the depth, openness, and vulnerability that men display in these discussions. Ask men, give them space and permission, and they will talk.

1.6 Men with Rheumatoid Arthritis (RA)

Rheumatoid arthritis is a type of long-term condition known as an auto-immune condition, which means the body's immune system mistakes its own healthy cells and tissues as foreign and attacks them. Rheumatoid arthritis causes painful, swollen, and stiff joints, and is often accompanied by fatigue. Symptoms can fluctuate on a daily basis and patients can experience unpredictable disease flares, which can be an exacerbation of existing symptoms and/or whole-body flu-like symptoms. If inflammation is uncontrolled it can lead to permanent joint damage and disability.

The cause of rheumatoid arthritis is unclear and there is currently no cure although treatment has improved to the point where remission is now a realistic treatment goal. The prevalence of rheumatoid arthritis varies globally from approximately 1% in the USA, 0.46% in Australasia, 0.44% in North America and Western Europe to as low as 0.16% in North Africa, Middle East, and Asia (Yip & Navarro-Millán, 2021). Rheumatoid arthritis is traditionally reported to affect predominantly white populations (around 75%). However, these figures reflect the ethnicity make-up of the countries that epidemiological data is most commonly collected from (in the UK and USA around 75% of the population are white). It is also possible that gaps in prevalence may reflect underdiagnosis due to health inequalities. Rheumatoid arthritis can begin at any age, but the peak age of onset is 30–60 years. Rheumatoid arthritis affects more women (around 70%) than men. Disease activity, structural damage, and joint deformities have been reported equally in men and women (using both subjective and objective measures). However, women report more disability than men. This could be due to physiological differences, scale psychometric bias (with the measures used in rheumatoid arthritis developed in study populations that reflect the larger number of women with the condition), or differences in symptom perception.

An unexpected finding in my PhD indicated that overall men were having a more negative experience of living with rheumatoid arthritis than women; they found it difficult to identify coping or self-management strategies that worked for them, and were uninterested in the psychosocial support available to them within rheumatology services (which generally took the form of talking groups where men were vastly outnumbered by women). This led to a post-doctoral fellowship, which comprised the following studies underpinning this book. These have been published elsewhere, but I will summarise them here to put this book into context:

A ***systematic literature review*** (Flurey et al., 2016a) to assess what is known about the psychosocial impact of rheumatoid arthritis on men; what is known about the coping and self-management styles of men with rheumatoid arthritis; and whether or not gender differences exist in these areas. The published literature (up to 2014) suggested that although men take longer to adjust and adapt to rheumatoid arthritis, women were more likely to report rheumatoid arthritis-related negative mood or distress. Men and women report differences in the way in which rheumatoid arthritis impacts their quality of life with it seeming to be more important for men's psychological wellbeing for them to remain in paid work than women. Women tend to report using a larger number and more diverse self-management strategies than men and receive more positive social support.

Focus groups with 22 men with rheumatoid arthritis were used to explore their experiences, coping styles, and support preferences (Flurey et al., 2016b). These male participants had a median age of 64 years (range 44–75 years), which is slightly older than the rheumatoid arthritis population (Dougados et al., 2014) and median disease duration of 9.5 years (range 2 months to 19 years). All participants were white British. I conducted six focus groups with small numbers to allow the men to feel comfortable discussing thoughts and feelings openly (Grogan & Richards, 2002). However, due to some non-attendance some focus groups were smaller than planned (2–5 participants in each).

I analysed the data using Braun & Clarke's thematic analysis (Braun & Clarke, 2021) and found three overarching themes relating to the way men experience and manage rheumatoid arthritis and the support they require:

1. "Challenges to masculinity", which described a reduction in strength and abilities that could lead to a loss of independence. It also included challenges to masculine identity and masculine roles, and the experience of losing power and control due to rheumatoid arthritis.
2. "Getting through life with RA" described how men coped with the condition. This included 'just getting on with it', seeking out information to try and understand their condition better, and for some men engaging in risk-taking behaviours such as drink and drug use or over exercising causing themselves pain and potential joint damage. Men also discussed withdrawing socially, which was due to no

longer being able to join in activities, or to protect loved ones from the emotional impact.
3. "Sources of support" tended not to include friends, as the men perceived them to lack understanding or support. Men discussed a preference for information giving sessions rather than discussion groups, but there was no agreement on whether these should be mixed gender or men only, or who should run the sessions.

Focus groups are useful for examining opinions and beliefs about an issue, whilst individual interviews are effective in exploring personal experiences (Molzahn et al., 2005) and their combination can provide complementary views of a studied phenomenon (Lambert & Loiselle, 2008). Thus, to explore both the breadth and depth of men's experiences of living with rheumatoid arthritis and its impact on masculine identity, I also invited a sub-set of focus group participants to take part in individual interviews.

One-to-one interviews with five men were used to explore the experience of being a man with rheumatoid arthritis and the impact on masculine identity in depth (Flurey et al., 2018b). Participants were invited to take part in the interviews to reflect a heterogeneous experience of life with rheumatoid arthritis, based on knowledge about the participants gained from the focus group discussions. Case studies of these five men identified three typologies for explaining the impact of rheumatoid arthritis on masculine identity: "Retaining hegemonic ideals of masculinity" described trying to hold on to activities and roles valued within hegemonic masculinity (e.g., sports activities, paid work) that they took part in before being diagnosed with rheumatoid arthritis. "Trying to renegotiate masculinity" described men who were no longer able to take part in certain masculine activities, which had been important to them before being diagnosed with rheumatoid arthritis. Dealing with this loss involved trying to find replacement activities or other ways of doing things and renegotiating how these adjustments fit into their perception of masculinity. Finally, "Rejection of hegemonic masculinity", which could be captured by Connell's subordinated masculinity, describes the experience of rejecting or being unconcerned about fitting in with the demands of hegemonic masculine ideals, which seemed to be both physically and psychologically protective for the men who fit this typology in these case studies.

The current book is predominantly concerned with the qualitative literature in considering how men discuss their experiences of long-term conditions. However, I will briefly mention that my Arthritis Research UK fellowship also included a Q-methodology study (this method was described in Sect. 1.4) and a national survey study. The Q-methodology study included 30 men with rheumatoid arthritis and found that some men take a pro-active approach to managing the impact of rheumatoid arthritis and find different ways of doing things, whilst others are determined to continue with their pre-rheumatoid arthritis lives and push themselves to carry on even if this causes them pain. They experience frustration and anger due to the impact of rheumatoid arthritis but internalise this rather than getting angry at the people around them (Flurey et al., 2016c).

My survey study included 280 men with rheumatoid arthritis across England and found that 43% of these men reported severe disease, less effective coping, and poor psychological status. Men tended to prefer practical support with a focus on expanding their knowledge about rheumatoid arthritis and how to manage it (Flurey et al., 2018a).

1.7 Men with Systemic Sclerosis (SSc)

Systemic sclerosis, also known as scleroderma, is an autoimmune condition that affects the skin and connective tissues (group of tissues in the body that maintain the form of the body and its organs). Systemic sclerosis causes the body to produce too much collagen, which causes hardening and tightening of the skin. Systemic sclerosis is a rare condition with a prevalence of roughly 0.002%, meaning it affects around 20 people in every 1 million. It affects around 2.5 million people worldwide. Systemic sclerosis can range from mild to severe and in some cases can be life threatening due to internal organ involvement. Individual symptoms can vary depending on the part of the body affected. The cause of systemic sclerosis is not known and there is currently no cure. Systemic sclerosis is more common in women compared to men, but the exact ratio between the sexes has varied widely in the reported literature. In general, the ratio between female and male systemic sclerosis patients is considered to be approximately 3:1 and has been reported as high as 7–8:1 (Hughes et al., 2020).

In general, men with systemic sclerosis have significantly reduced survival rates than women and report more severe disease (Hughes et al., 2020). Rheumatologists have told me they experience a 'heart sink' when diagnosing men with systemic sclerosis due to these survival rates and were keen to better understand how to support men. This led to a focus group study to explore the experiences of men with systemic sclerosis; how it impacts their lives; how men currently cope with and manage systemic sclerosis; and their preferences for support (Flurey et al., 2022).

Twenty-five men with systemic sclerosis from the UK and USA participated with a mean age of 58 years (range 37–78 years), and mean disease duration of 8 years (range 1–29 years). The majority of were White (76%), married (76%), and retired (40%), with education levels ranging from elementary to post-graduate. Seven focus groups (three USA, four UK) were conducted with three to six participants in each to allow the men to feel comfortable discussing thoughts and feelings openly. Three overarching themes and one underpinning theme were identified:

"Impact of SSc on masculinity" included the impact of systemic sclerosis on masculine roles and activities. Men reported sex, intimacy, and erectile dysfunction as salient issues that weren't generally addressed by their clinicians. They also experienced challenges to their masculine self-image due to weight and muscle loss affecting how their bodies looked and felt. "Dealing with SSc" meant always being prepared through planning ahead for anticipated difficulties. The men became or aimed to become experts in systemic sclerosis through seeking out information from various sources, and they made conscious decisions about balancing their priorities between responsibilities, maintaining activities that mattered to them, and managing their symptoms. Whilst they didn't always prioritise symptom management this seemed to be through calculated risks rather than recklessness. "Support for living with SSc" included men being selective in who they talked to about systemic sclerosis and the level and nature of their disclosure. These men would (reluctantly) accept help as they didn't always have a choice due to the severity of their condition. Underpinning these experiences was 'facing an uncertain future' due to the life-limiting nature of the condition. Some men preferred not to focus on an unpredictable future, and others experienced ongoing worries about disease progression.

1.8 Searching the Men with Long-Term Conditions Literature

My studies in rheumatoid arthritis and systemic sclerosis have provided a starting point and framework for structuring this book. Whilst these conditions differ in their severity and clinical manifestation, they are both autoimmune rheumatic diseases that have a higher prevalence in women than men. To fully inform a book on men with long-term conditions it has therefore been crucial to look to the wider literature.

To do this, I searched MEDLINE, CINAHL, AMED, and PsychInfo databases for qualitative, psychosocial literature on men with long-term conditions. This was to ensure I had oversight of the full existing body of qualitative literature on men with long-term conditions. However, this book is not intended as a systematic literature review. It is not possible to include all this literature in one book in a meaningful way and I have made pragmatic decisions for inclusion.

For example, due to the wealth of studies on men with prostate cancer I have had to be particularly selective to avoid this condition dominating the book and have been unable to include all of these studies. However, the voices of men with prostate cancer still feature in almost every chapter. I have aimed to include the full range of long-term conditions I could find in the literature. In conditions with particularly limited literature, I have included every study I could find, whilst some conditions may not be reported on at all due to being unable to find relevant literature. I have predominantly included studies that focus solely on men unless gender differences or men's experiences have been particularly highlighted and are apparent from the included data.

As you will see from the demographics in my above studies, I am acutely aware of the lack of diversity in my own participant populations. My focus groups on men with systemic sclerosis included some ethnic diversity, and both studies included men who disclosed being gay during the focus group discussions. However, none of my studies explicitly focused on how these men's experiences may differ and there were insufficient participants to make any inferences from their narratives. Thus, I have made a concerted effort to include all studies I could find on men from other countries, and from a range of ethnicities and sexualities. Literature on experiences of men with long-term conditions from marginalised groups is sparse, particularly on men who identify as LGBTQIA+. This is a gap that needs filling in future research to better inform our understanding and the design of care and support provision for men.

1.9 Book Structure

The book will be divided into the following chapters, which reflect broad categories of key issues in relation to men living with long-term conditions.

Chapter 2, **'Impact on Masculine Roles and Activities'**, explores the way men talk about the impact of long-term conditions on their daily and valued life activities. I discuss the effect long-term conditions can have on men's sense of masculinity including the impact on traditionally masculine roles, activities, and their capacity for self-reliance. Men's self-worth and masculinity can be intricately linked to their occupational status and in this chapter, I discuss the real or implied pressure men can feel to fulfil a bread-winner role. This chapter also includes the way long-term conditions impact men's family roles.

Chapter 3, **'Mental Wellbeing'**, includes the way men talk about mental health, the value they often place on being 'mentally strong', and challenges the social narrative that 'men don't cry'. In this chapter I go beyond the physical long-term conditions literature and draw on the mental health literature particularly in depression and anxiety to help understand and contextualise the experiences of men with physical conditions. I explore the ways that men do open up with each other about emotional impact, whilst sometimes masking the full impact from those closest to them. The chapter finishes with what can be learnt from Bristol-based charity Talk Club and their strategies for encouraging men to talk about what they term 'mental fitness'.

Chapter 4, **'Self-Image and Body Image'**, explores the way men discuss the impact of illness on their self-image and body image. This includes the way men discuss visible differences or physical changes to their bodies such as loss of muscle mass or hair loss. This also includes a consideration of the way men talk about dealing with the impact to their self-image and body image, which can be through attempts to hide visible signs of their condition or rejecting being treated in a way that reinforces a negative self-image.

Chapter 5, **'Sex and intimacy'** explores the way men talk about the impact of illness on sex and intimacy. This covers not only erectile dysfunction but also barriers to intimacy caused by physical symptoms. I discuss how men's concerns go beyond sexual satisfaction to the impact on their partner's satisfaction, romantic relationships, and confidence. The chapter finishes with an exploration of how men approach the topic of sex and intimacy, the language they use, and who they feel most comfortable talking to.

From *la petite mort* to **'Mortality'**, **Chapter 6** explores the way men with long-term conditions talk about their mortality. This includes how the threat of mortality can act as a wake-up call to change health behaviours, and focuses on the issues men worry about when living with a life-limiting condition. The responsibility to be the protector and provider of the family often remains at the forefront for men, even when faced with their mortality. I also discuss the approach men take to talking about death from the dark humour used to deal with discussing difficult topics to the raw honesty about their fears of dying.

Chapter 7, **'Coping and Self-Management'**, focuses on the way men talk about coping and self-management for long-term conditions. This includes how men begin to reclaim the control lost due to illness through taking responsibility for their disease management and becoming experts in their condition. Many men discuss the importance of keeping going despite limitations imposed by illness, and this chapter covers the various creative ways they employ to manage this. Whilst public narratives suggest men don't talk about their health, in this chapter I discuss how men will engage in selective disclosure with trusted others. This chapter also covers risk-taking in the context of a long-term condition, and I discuss how men with long-term conditions may take calculated rather than reckless risks in managing their health. Finally, this covers how men discuss acceptance of their condition, with some men redefining their masculinity to support effective coping.

Chapter 8, **'Help-Seeking'**, focuses on men's help-seeking or health-seeking behaviours for long-term conditions. I start by challenging the prevailing public narrative that men are worse than women at seeking medical help, suggesting that men and women may have different reasons for delaying help-seeking. I explore how men talk about engagement with healthcare services, their motivations for seeking help, and reasons for delaying. Finally, I consider ways to encourage men to seek help sooner.

Chapter 9, **'Support'**, focuses on the ways men discuss preferring to receive and access support and who they choose to open up to. I discuss what men want from their clinical team, whether male-only support services are preferred, and the role of family and peer support. This chapter also includes what works for men in designing support services in terms of the setting, facilitating communication, and providing a clear purpose. This chapter finishes with an overview of two exemplar interventions for supporting men (Men's Sheds and Football Fans in Training).

Chapter 10, **'Men Talking in Metaphors'**, considers the metaphors men use in talking about their health. Whilst men are often cited as using battle metaphors to talk about illness, this chapter considers that this may not be a solely male way of talking about illness and offers other examples of metaphors men use to talk about long-term conditions. This includes illness as an unpredictable predator, highlighting a loss of power and control; and the body as a machine, using technology metaphors to make sense of their condition. Overall, men's metaphors often capture salient aspects of their condition and provide an insight into imagery through language that may be helpful in talking to men about long-term conditions.

Chapter 11, 'Tips for Supporting Men', summarises the key practical learning points that can be used in an applied context. It draws the contents of this book together in the form of top tips for some of the key players involved in supporting men with long-term conditions. This includes ten tips for healthcare professionals working with men with long-term conditions, ten tips for researchers looking to engage men in research, and ten tips for those developing support services for men.

Glossary of long-term conditions: In this introduction chapter I have described rheumatoid arthritis and systemic sclerosis, and throughout the book I will refer to a number of other long-term conditions from the literature. To help the flow of the book I won't define and describe each long-term condition as it arises, so a summary of each included long-term condition can be found in a glossary at the end of this book.

A note on presentations of quotes throughout: For quotes from my own data, I have included participants' age, condition, and ethnicity (n.b. data on patients' demographics were missing from one site for the systemic sclerosis focus groups). Where possible, I have included this for quotes from the wider literature, but this was not always available from the original papers. Where ethnicity was missing I have included the country participants were recruited from. For quotes from my own data, where these have been previously published either in part or in full (often the quotes presented in the book are fuller than the paper) I have cited the paper where these are originally published (to acknowledge copyright).

1.10 Summary

Men are more likely to die prematurely than women at all ages, and for all causes. Whilst social narratives tell us men are bad for their own health, it is increasingly acknowledged that men are under-served by health services. Men need their own health strategy, and this includes providing tailored care and support for men with long-term conditions. This book will use my own research in men with rheumatoid arthritis and systemic sclerosis as a basis to explore the wider literature on men with long-term conditions and discuss how men talk about their health, and their experiences of the physical and emotional impact of living with a long-term condition. It will include how men cope and self-manage, and provide implications for practice and suggestions for how to support men using examples from existing successful initiatives. I hope this book will be of use to healthcare professionals, researchers, policymakers—and anyone who is a man or who knows a man.

References

Aurita, N., & Huda, M. (2018). Hierarchy of masculinities in George R.R. Martin's A Game of Thrones. In *Proceedings of The1st International Conference on Recent Innovations*, 614–621.

Braun, V., & Clarke, V. (2021). *Thematic analysis: A practical guide*. SAGE.

Broom, A., & Cavenagh, J. (2010). Masculinity, moralities and being cared for: An exploration of experiences of living and dying in a hospice. *Social Science & Medicine, 71*(5), 869–876. https://doi.org/10.1016/J.SOCSCIMED.2010.05.026

Connell, R. W. (2005). *Masculinities* (2nd ed.). University of California Press.

Connell, R. W., & Messerschmidt, J. W. (2005). Hegemonic masculinity rethinking the concept. *Gender & Society, 19*(6), 829–859.

Courtenay, W. H. (2000). Constructions of masculinity and their influence on men's well-being: A theory of gender and health. *Social Science & Medicine, 50*(10), 1385–1401.

del Mar García-Calvente, M., Hidalgo-Ruzzante, N., del Río-Lozano, M., Marcos-Marcos, J., Martínez-Morante, E., Maroto-Navarro, G., Mateo-Rodríguez, I., & Gil-García, E. (2012). Exhausted women, tough men: A qualitative study on gender differences in health, vulnerability and coping with illness in Spain. *Sociology of Health & Illness, 16.*

Department of Health. (2012). *Long-term conditions compendium of Information: 3rd edition.*

Dougados, M., Soubrier, M., Antunez, A., Balint, P., Balsa, A., Buch, M. H., et al. (2014). Prevalence of comorbidities in rheumatoid arthritis and evaluation of their monitoring: Results of an international, cross-sectional study (COMORA). *Annals of the Rheumatic Diseases, 73*(1), 62–68. https://doi.org/10.1136/annrheumdis-2013-204223

Equality Act, c. 15 (2010). https://www.legislation.gov.uk/ukpga/2010/15/contents

Flurey, C., Hewlett, S., Rodham, K., White, A., Noddings, R., & Kirwan, J. (2016a). Men, rheumatoid arthritis, psychosocial impact and self-management:

A narrative review. *Journal of Health Psychology, 21*(10), 2168–2182. https://doi.org/1359105315572452

Flurey, C., Hewlett, S., Rodham, K., White, A., Noddings, R., & Kirwan, J. (2016b). "You obviously just have to put on a brave face": A qualitative study of the experiences and coping styles of men with rheumatoid arthritis. *Arthritis Care & Research, 69*(3), 330–337.

Flurey, C., Hewlett, S., Rodham, K., White, A., Noddings, R., & Kirwan, J. R. (2016c). Identifying different typologies of experiences and coping strategies in men with rheumatoid arthritis: A Q-methodology study. *BMJ Open, 6*(10), e012051. https://doi.org/10.1136/bmjopen-2016-012051

Flurey, C., Hewlett, S., Rodham, K., White, A., Noddings, R., & Kirwan, J. R. (2018a). Coping strategies, psychological impact and support preferences of men with rheumatoid arthritis: A multicentre survey. *Arthritis Care & Research, 70*(6), 851–860.

Flurey, C., Morris, M., Pollock, J., Richards, P., Hughes, R., & Hewlett, S. (2014a). Fluctuating balances: A Q-methodology study of flare help-seeking behaviours and different experiences of daily life in Rheumatoid Arthritis. *BMC Musculoskeletal Disorders, 15*, 364.

Flurey, C., Pauling, J. D., Saketkoo, L. A., Denton, C. P., Galdas, P., Khanna, D., Williams, A., & Hughes, M. (2022). 'I turned in my man card': A qualitative study of the experiences, coping styles and support needs of men with systemic sclerosis. *Rheumatology, 62*(6), 2160–2167. https://doi.org/10.1093/RHEUMATOLOGY/KEAC585

Flurey, C., White, A., Rodham, K., Kirwan, J., Noddings, R., & Hewlett, S. (2018b). 'Everyone assumes a man to be quite strong': Men, masculinity and rheumatoid arthritis: A case-study approach. *Sociology of Health & Illness, 40*(1), 115–129.

Freeman, A., Mergl, R., Kohls, E., Székely, A., Gusmao, R., Arensman, E., Koburger, N., Hegerl, U., & Rummel-Kluge, C. (2017). A cross-national study on gender differences in suicide intent. *BMC Psychiatry, 17*(1), 1–11. https://doi.org/10.1186/S12888-017-1398-8

Frosh, S., Phoenix, A., & Pattman, R. (2002). *Young Masculinities.* Palgrave Macmillan.

Galdas, P., Darwin, Z., Kidd, L., Blickem, C., McPherson, K., Hunt, K., Bower, P., Gilbody, S., & Richardson, G. (2014). The accessibility and acceptability of self-management support interventions for men with long term conditions: A systematic review and meta-synthesis of qualitative studies. *BMC Public Health, 14*(1), 1230.

Galdas, P., Fell, J., Bower, P., Kidd, L., Blickem, C., McPherson, K., Hunt, K., Gilbody, S., & Richardson, G. (2015). The effectiveness of self-management support interventions for men with long-term conditions: A systematic review and meta-analysis. *BMJ Open, 5*(e006620). https://doi.org/10.1136/bmjopen-2014-006620

Gough, B., Robertson, S., & Luck, H. (2021). Engendered expressions of anxiety: Men's emotional communications with women and other men. *Frontiers in Sociology, 6*. https://doi.org/10.3389/FSOC.2021.697356
Grogan, S., & Richards, H. (2002). Body image. *Men and Masculinities, 4*(3), 219–232.
Hughes, M., Pauling, J. D., Armstrong-James, L., Denton, C. P., Galdas, P., & Flurey, C. (2020). Gender-related differences in systemic sclerosis. In *Autoimmunity Reviews* (Vol. 19, Issue 4, p. 102494). Elsevier B.V. https://doi.org/10.1016/j.autrev.2020.102494
Lambert, S. D., & Loiselle, C. G. (2008). Combining individual interviews and focus groups to enhance data richness. *Journal of Advanced Nursing, 62*(2), 228–237.
McCaughan, E., Prue, G., Parahoo, K., McIlfatrick, S., & McKenna, H. (2011). Exploring and comparing the experience and coping behaviour of men and women with colorectal cancer at diagnosis and during surgery. *Journal of Advanced Nursing, 67*(7), 1591–1600.
McCormack, M., & Anderson, E. (2010). "It's just not acceptable any more": The erosion of homophobia and the softening of masculinity at an English sixth form. *Sociology, 44*(5), 843–859. https://doi.org/10.1177/0038038510375734
Molzahn, A. E., Starzomski, R., McDonald, M., & O'Loughlin, C. (2005). Chinese Canadian beliefs toward organ donation. *Qualitative Health Research, 15*(1), 82–98.
Oliffe, J., & Mróz, L. (2005). Men interviewing men about health and illness: Ten lessons learned. *The Journal of Men's Health & Gender, 2*(2), 257–260.
Richards, H., & Emslie, C. (2000). The 'doctor' or the 'girl from the university'? Considering the influence of professional roles on qualitative interviewing. *Family Practice, 17*(1), 71–75.
Schwalbe, M., & Wolkomir, M. (2001). The masculine self as problem and resource in interview studies of men. *Men and Masculinities, 4*(1), 90–103.
Watts, S., & Stenner, P. (2012). *Doing Q methodological research: Theory, method and interpretation*. Sage.
White, A., De Sousa, B., De Visser, R., Hogston, R., Madsen, S. A., Makara, P., McKee, M., Raine, G., Richardson, N., & Clarke, N. (2011). Men's health in Europe. *Journal of Men's Health, 8*(3), 192–201.
Witty, K., Branney, P., Bullen, K., White, A., Evans, J., & Eardley, I. (2014). Engaging men with penile cancer in qualitative research: Reflections from an interview-based study. *Nurse Researcher, 21*(3), 13–19.
Yip, K., & Navarro-Millán, I. (2021). Racial, ethnic, and healthcare disparities in rheumatoid arthritis. *Current Opinion in Rheumatology, 33*(2), 117–121. https://doi.org/10.1097/BOR.0000000000000782

CHAPTER 2

Impact on Masculine Roles and Activities

"You're supposed to be the man about the house"

Hegemonic masculinity (as described in Chap. 1) is a concept that relates to the current most prized way of being a man in a particular locale. Findings throughout the literature conclude that illness can threaten hegemonic masculine ideals such as stoicism, self-reliance, and being in control (Connell, 2005). This can cause men to feel worried about "*standing out from the herd*" (O'Brien et al., 2007): distinct from other men as they are unable to 'perform' masculinity in different contexts in ways they have been accustomed to at other times in their adult life.

2.1 Negotiating Loss of Power and Control

Strength is commonly thought of as a cornerstone of masculinity, whether physical or emotional, and many of the men throughout my studies and the wider literature described their symptoms in relation to the impact they had on their strength: "*It saps your strength*" (Robert, rheumatoid arthritis). This reduction in physical strength was described as a key loss, which challenged their feelings of self-worth and sense of competence. Being unable to keep up with or match up to the strength and abilities of other men was often experienced as humiliating:

C. Flurey, *Talking Men's Health*,
https://doi.org/10.1007/978-3-031-62593-0_2

The lads laugh at me because I used to be like them shoot up trees hang off scaffolding, that nimble, that's what breast cancer did to me, from that to this. (Darren, breast cancer, UK) (Quincey et al., 2021)

It's sort of humiliating really. The things I used to do which I can't. Now that I know I'm paying other people to do (them) and stand by and watch some other bloke do it. (Participant 7, 55yrs, osteoporosis, UK) (Minns Lowe et al., 2019)

A handshake is a key social interaction in Western contexts that works to reinforce masculine ideals of what it means to be dominant, professional, and in control. Many men who experienced issues with their hands due to a long-term condition highlighted their frustrations with this common interaction. Handshakes are such an important element of non-verbal communication in a business setting that those who were unable to effectively shake hands discussed feeling their position weakened:

We needed to have a hard conversation and so the last thing I wanted was to feel weak by spearing the guy in the hand and having to apologise to him in the first two seconds. (Patient B, 46yrs, rheumatoid arthritis, UK) (Lack et al., 2011)

In social settings, men often felt anger or resentment towards those who exerted their power through a firm gripped handshake due to the pain they caused, and some suggested they get around this by swerving a handshake in favour of a hug or kiss:

Ron	*And you greet one another, shake hands, cor dear, and some of them when they shook my hand it was like argh. Do you know what I mean? It was like that, you wouldn't tell anybody about it, and you say, err, you just felt like saying 'next time you do that mate I'm going to give you what for' [laughs].*
Frank	*Bop you on the nose [laughs]*
Ron	*Kick you on the leg like, you know.*
Edward	*I used to be like it, and I got to the stage where I actually don't shake hands anymore, I don't put my hand out, which is not me.*
Ron	*I go for the cheek first.*
Edward	*I was going to say I'm more inclined to give someone a hug. (Focus group of men with rheumatoid arthritis, UK)*

Men often discussed "*battling through*" their symptoms as much as possible to avoid having to show "*weakness*" in front of others. However, this can have consequences in exacerbating their symptoms such as causing themselves more pain, or even long-term damage. Depending on the severity or progression of the long-term condition it wasn't always possible to 'battle through':

Travis	*So, it's frustrating like you said, it's frustrating and, you know, like most men they don't want to show, you know, like you can't do anything.*
Jorge	*Weakness.*
Travis	*Weakness, good word, so you battle through it [coughs] you know, every day but recently, er, in the last couple of years it has affected my lungs which is really, er, taking a toll on me because now it went from just being frustrated and to the point where I just can't do it, you know, I just can't do it.*
	(Focus group of men with systemic sclerosis, USA)

Loss of control due to a body that no longer behaves as expected or desired was a commonly occurring issue for men with long-term conditions, which challenged their sense of masculinity. This experience of losing control differed across conditions. Some experienced a loss of control over the planning and direction of day-to-day life due to unpredictable fluctuations in symptoms such as pain and fatigue: "*You can't do something that you said to yourself the day before I'll do*" (George, rheumatoid arthritis). Whereas those who lived with symptoms of bladder or bowel incontinence faced a much more direct experience of loss of control, which Roger (below) describes as eroding his masculinity. He also uses language such as "*weak*" and "*fail*", further illustrating decreasing self-esteem:

> *Getting to the toilet in time. You know, it's a simple thing but it erodes your masculinity a little bit doesn't it. You know. So why I wear white trousers I dunno. Simple things like that, if you happen to be weak, it takes a hell of a lot of bladder control. I can just about make it, but sometimes you fail. It doesn't do anything for your masculinity does it. (Roger, 55yrs, Parkinson's disease, UK)* (Gibson & Kierans, 2017)

In addition to experiencing loss of control over their lives due to the symptoms associated with long-term conditions, men also discussed a lack of control over their disease progression. Healthcare professionals could amplify or diminish these feelings of loss of control through their approaches. It's widely accepted that the balance of power between patients and healthcare professionals can be tricky to negotiate (Khazen, 2022). When men felt healthcare professionals didn't believe them, dismissed or diminished their concerns, didn't treat them with care, or blamed them for their condition they described being left feeling helpless, which sometimes triggered feelings of anger and aggression:

Will *He [doctor] just yanked my finger and I nearly lumped him straight through the wall. 'Don't you ever do that to me again.' I said, you know, that hurt. And I, I really … I did threaten him. And another fellow came along, he said, 'oh, we'll have none of that'. I said 'well, what about him? Can't you …' they know that I've got something wrong with my hands and yet he catches hold of it like that.*

John *I had a similar problem when I had x-rays done at first, I think it was hands, chest and feet erm, I was leaning against the x-ray plate, and this nurse …*

Will *Tried to yank your arm behind your back.*

John *Just dragged my arms back and pulled. … It was so painful, and I said to her, 'for God's sake, do you know what I've got and why I'm …' I couldn't believe she'd do that.*

Will *Yes, they did the same to me with my shoulders, they tried to yank … they said 'put your arms behind your back', so I'm going like this, and she goes, 'no, like this'. Oh, fwor … you know, my language was not very polite and I don't think she's ever forgiven me. But who cares, she shouldn't do that, no one should do that to you.*
(Focus group of men with rheumatoid arthritis, UK)

Many men appreciated efforts by healthcare professionals to reduce the power imbalance in consultations. For some men, male clinicians may hold the ability to confer or deny masculine status through their approach, and many men valued clinicians who honoured their masculine status. At the very least men sought basic human kindness and compassion, and to be treated respectfully by their clinical team:

> *He's [rheumatologist] really down at your level isn't he, he's a man's man … he's just a bloke. (Ron, 60yrs, rheumatoid arthritis, White British)* (Flurey et al., 2016b)

> *The nurses are different ... they have this compassion in them ... [...] when they hear that you have this illness, they kind of put the professional role aside and the human person steps in. ... But when you get to see the male doctors ... their attitude is different ... much more negative ... they belittle the symptoms, say that it's all in the head and so on. ... It is so fucking infuriating! (Steve, mid-20s, fibromyalgia, Norway)* (Sallinen et al., 2019)

Men deal with loss of control due to long-term conditions in various ways. Some discussed choosing avoidance or resigning themselves to a fatalistic outlook of their condition being beyond their control ("*[T]here is no control here [...] it's out of my control*" P4, advanced prostate cancer (Stapleton & Pattison, 2014)). Others focused on self-managing the parts of their condition they did have control over, or highly valued and protected the areas of their lives where they could exert control (self-management and coping strategies are discussed further in Chap. 7). My Q-methodology study with men with rheumatoid arthritis (see Chap. 1) found that those men who were able to retain control in some areas of their lives (e.g., autonomy at work) were better able to accept a certain amount of loss of control due to rheumatoid arthritis than others (Flurey et al., 2016c). Paul explains the importance to him of shooting as a hobby as it enables him to demonstrate his ability to take control:

> *[T]hat's one of my coping strategies ... shooting for me it's control ... when I shoot, I pride myself on hitting what I'm aiming at and having to be totally controlled under those circumstances. (Paul, breast cancer, UK)* (Quincey et al., 2021)

2.2 Self-reliance and Independence

For many men, long-term conditions affect their ability to be self-reliant or independent. For some this is a particularly marked impact due to needing help with self-care tasks such as washing and dressing. As illustrated by Jacob and Boat (below) many of the men praised the patience and care of their spouses or partners but discussed the emotional impact of having to be dependent on them. Having to receive help for basic care tasks was seen as infantilising or a regression to childhood. Boat describes how he perceives his status in the family as diminished due to needing this support. In many African cultures, masculinity is associated with status, dignity, independence, and superiority (Salifu et al., 2023). So, this impact on men's social status due to a loss of self-reliance and independence could have a particularly marked impact on African men's sense of masculinity and self-worth:

> *Do you know how it feels to have your wife to put your socks your shoes, help you put your underwears on, got to help you to get in the bath tub, you know, what I mean, that, that, you know, that hurts. You know, that really do hurt, but I thank God for her, 'cause if I didn't have her, I'd probably have to go to a nursing home. (Jacob, 62yrs, systemic sclerosis, African American)* (Flurey et al., 2022)

> *[N]ow the whole situation is like moving straight from the head of the family to the tail. Because when one is unable to do something for himself [care], he becomes like a child, needing to be cared for. (Boat, prostate cancer, Ghanaian)* (Salifu et al., 2023)

The following focus group interaction between three men with rheumatoid arthritis demonstrates the emotional toll of losing self-reliance and independence. This loss of being able to rely on their bodies is experienced as a loss of independence, a loss of dignity, it's "*soul destroying*". Despite the common narrative that men don't cry, David freely shares that he "*was in tears*" with the other men in the group who instantly respond by relating their own experiences, legitimising his reaction. Tears of frustration due to physical limitations experienced by the rest of the group may be an example of expressing 'manly emotion' (Warner & Shields, 2007). This may be permissible amongst other men in the same way that it may be acceptable for men to cry when their favourite football team loses:

David *I was in tears on the garage floor because I'd got a drill and I couldn't get up off the floor. Unbelievable. And same thing, I went to get out of a chair once, couldn't get out of the chair. I thought, oh, all right, I'll get on the floor, get on my knees, pick myself up. No, wouldn't happen. Getting the same thing, about an hour before I could get up, couldn't believe it.*

James *One of the worst things you can do, when you've got it bad, is get down on your knees. 'Cos you can't get up. Without some support somewhere you can't get up.*

David *That's right. And even then, I couldn't get up. I didn't have the strength in my knees to … couldn't believe it.*

James *It sounds funny, but it's so soul destroying because what it does, it takes away your self … you're sort of dependent ….*
Robert *Yeh, your dignity.*
James *Your own ability to look after … just your basic life, you know what I mean?*
(Focus group of men with rheumatoid arthritis, UK)

Amongst limitations due to long-term conditions, it was often important for men to express the things that they were still able to do for themselves. For example, Dafydd who has Parkinson's disease, which can restrict dexterous, skilful work due to tremors, describes how he retained the skill of wiring a plug:

> *It was wiring a plug, that's the simplest thing in the world, wiring a plug. But because of the way I couldn't grip properly, I had to find all sorts of ways of manipulating the screwdriver, very frustrating. Over the years I think I improved, I can still put a wire in a plug, purely and simply because of what I've learnt. What I've learnt is that the body, and the brain, can be trained to organise a job, to do it in a different way. (Dafydd, 73yrs, Parkinson's disease, UK)* (Gibson & Kierans, 2017)

Independence is highly valued by people across long-term conditions, and not limited to men. It may be assumed that men would place higher expectations on themselves for what constitutes retaining their independence. However, the below quote from Caitlin, explaining what independence means to her from one of my focus groups (to develop an outcome measure for independence), demonstrates that women also hold themselves to high standards for physical abilities:

> *I don't need someone else around to help out with anything. Um, you know, even opening stuff or, um, like for me in the winter shovelling snow kind of a thing. (Caitlin, rheumatoid arthritis, Canadian)*

However, the added layer for men seems to be that loss of independence challenges their masculine status. This seemed particularly salient when men had to ask for help with things that were traditionally seen as a marker of strength such as being able to open a tight lid on a jar or bottle. As the quote from Steve demonstrates, having to ask for help from their wives ('the weaker sex') served as an unwelcome reminder of their loss of strength. Ted explains that when asking other men for help he would make a self-deprecating joke. He explains the reason for this as making the other person feel comfortable, but humour can also be protective in mocking ourselves before someone else does:

> *Until I got it, I thought I was invincible and then all of a sudden I've got my missus opening jars for me and it's just like, 'good grief!' you know. When you're supposed to be the man about the house. (Steve, 44yrs rheumatoid arthritis, White British)*

> *I say that as a joke, in a way to just, you know, 'cause I understand as a man asking somebody to open your bottle of water it can be embarrassing. It doesn't bother me at all, but I want them to feel comfortable too, so I make a joke about it. I just say 'here, I turned in my man card, open this for me' and we all laugh and move on. (Ted, 68yrs, systemic sclerosis, White American)*

2.3 Impact on Social Activities

For people with long-term conditions loss of independence extends to being able to take part in social or valued activities. For many men, social connection is built and sustained through engagement in shared activities. Thus, when they are no longer able to engage in these shared activities, they can begin to lose their social support networks. Men discussed withdrawing from social interactions for a variety of reasons such as embarrassment (e.g., due to the potential for incontinence (Alexis & Worsley, 2018)), or being unable to engage in the masculine drinking culture of their friendship group due to restrictions of their medication:

> *With the medication that I've been on over the last couple of years erm, it's not been advisable for me to even risk a small drink, so I gave up going to pubs completely because I just didn't feel right going into a pub and having soft drinks. (Mike, 60yrs, rheumatoid arthritis, White British)* (Flurey et al., 2016b)

Engaging in physical activities were often off limits or restricted due to pain and disability. Many of the men discussed preferring to give up on activities altogether rather than engage in a limited version of the activity or perform it to a lesser extent. As Scott describes below, whilst he was concerned that playing volleyball might cause him pain, he was equally worried that his performance would fall short of the standards he sets himself. He chooses to depart from masculine ideals of stoicism and competitiveness rather than risk a potentially humiliating public challenge to his competence:

> *Some of my friends wanted to play volleyball and they're like, 'well let's go and play', and I was like 'no, I don't really want to try that', and they were like, 'why not? Just try …' I'm like, 'well, it's hard to explain but one I might hurt myself, two it might just be so embarrassing that I'm not going to be happy with it', right, it's like, you know, and I can just tell they couldn't really understand like, like how can it be that bad. I was like 'well I don't know how to explain it to you'. (Scott, 43yrs, systemic sclerosis, White American)*

David (below) describes the emotional impact of being left out by his friendship group when his rheumatoid arthritis was too uncontrolled to enable him to join in. You can see by my follow-up question as the interviewer that I was surprised (and doing my best to hide indignance) that his friends left to have fun without him, perhaps applying female friendship codes where the activity would likely have been changed to something less physically demanding. However, for some male friendships the shared planned activity can be the central focus rather than the time spent together, meaning being unable to participate can mean being left behind:

David *The worst time … the worst time it affected me was when it caught on really bad in the beginning and I had a thing booked up to go to the Isle of Man TT [Tourist Trophy: motorcycle racing event], which is what I always wanted to do, and it come on, I thought what am I going to do. I was making clutch levers and break levers that was longer so I could put more leverage on and stuff like this. And er, I went out one day and er, all my mates went out on their bikes and … and I just couldn't go out the hotel. I was so bad I just had to sit in the hotel, and there was nothing more frustrating for me, and I was sat at the hotel and all my mates was whizzing round Douglas prom[enade] on their bikes. Oh, I was gutted.*

CF *Did any of them stay back with you?*

David *Well, no, I told them to … they'd have stayed there but I said no, you go on out, you know, didn't want to be that selfish. But er, it was pfft, depressing is a word doesn't come near how I felt that day. (58yrs, rheumatoid arthritis, White British)*

2.4 The Role of 'Breadwinner'

In many cultures, productivity and the role of the 'breadwinner' (main earner in the household) are defining features of dominant masculine ideals. These are constantly reinforced through societal expectations and the media (Vigorito & Curry, 1998). For men in (heterosexual) relationships, occupational status and income can be important for eliciting deference or respect from their partners (Schrock & Schwalbe, 2009), which may be even more important to them when their masculinity feels threatened by life with a long-term condition. However, this can also be experienced as a burden, with men in the breadwinner role feeling they have no choice but to continue working to meet their family's financial commitments:

CF *Did you ever consider giving up work when you …*
Mark *I did when I was really bad but then when you have got you know … my daughter was in university and my son was still at school you haven't really got a lot of choice but to carry on, even to go through the pain, loads of painkillers and carry on. (49yrs, rheumatoid arthritis, White British)*

> *When I look at my children I think I may die any moment and who will raise those children? … I have to save and make more effort to fulfil their needs until they grow up. (Male participant, cardiovascular disease, Arabic)* (Donnelly et al., 2019)

Some men who were no longer able to work tried to compensate for this by taking on domestic roles within the home. However, as the following quote from Paul demonstrates they often felt that this fell short, and they were failing to fulfil a role that was expected of them:

> *I clean the house, I do the chores to compensate […] but even when she [wife] comes through the door at five o'clock there's like a resentment there. Not, not malicious resentment, she can't help herself, like where's my bloke he should be doing his bit too, and I want to do my bit. I've proudly done my bit for 30 years of my life, I've worked 30 years of my life properly, so all of a sudden someone's put the brakes on. (Paul, 52yrs, systemic sclerosis, White British)*

For single men, occupation and income can be important for demonstrating worth to a potential partner. In heterosexual relationships, whilst successful women may no longer be seeking a man who can wholly provide for them, they still often desire a man who can hold his own financially to match their lifestyle. In same sex relationships, paid work and household tasks tend to be more equally divided between the couple (Bauer, 2016; Jaspers & Verbakel, 2013), which may create its own pressure for men to match up to their potential partner's financial worth. However, the literature on gay men with long-term conditions is sparse, and one particular gap is the impact of long-term conditions on single gay men. The below quote demonstrates the worries felt by single men in whether they will be able to have a family, as they question the value they would bring to a potential relationship:

> *I want that life a lot …with the wife and the kids and the grandkids and the extended family … how on earth do I get that, because to support a family you need like a good job, you need money, you need a good career. (Barth syndrome, USA)* (Mazar & Moorman, 2021)

Men with long-term conditions throughout the literature defined their masculinity and self-worth according to their work status. Wade (below) is living with a life-limiting condition (systemic sclerosis) and experienced a cardiac arrest. His poignant quote explains that although he's grateful to be alive and values his family, his perceived lack of purpose through not having a job or being the main wage earner leaves him doubting his value:

> *Before scleroderma, like you I was the breadwinner, I made the money and of course my wife works also, so we both do, but I made the most money and now that I'm disabled I mean I do have disability insurance, I do have an income but now my wife, she retired and she went back to work [laughs] and now she is the primary, she makes more money than me. Not that that bothers me, but I feel my self-worth, what do I do, I don't do anything anymore, besides live. I don't have a job anymore. And I try, it's all about my health and I go to [city] every three months for check-ups and it's all about my health but I, what am I living for, what's there to live for. I'm very fortunate and I'm very grateful and I'm happy. … My organs are working, I have a granddaughter which I was not supposed to be here for and so I'm holding a granddaughter now and it's wonderful, but still, I just. … And it's not a pity party, I'm not trying to feel sorry for myself it's just I ask myself, what am I here for? (Wade, 61yrs, systemic sclerosis, White American)*

Many men prioritised remaining in paid work over their own health. Some talked proudly of declining their doctor's offers to sign them off work citing the importance of having a purpose to keep them motivated. For many men, remaining in paid work was particularly important for preserving their status and positioning themselves as masculine:

> *[B]ut I need to earn my money, I mean you are already taking my manliness away, taking everything away from me, you are stripping me bit by bit, right, I just thought no … cost what it will cost, I have to take charge of my life, I have to be looked up to again as a man. (Mr Nelson, prostate cancer, Black Caribbean)* (Bamidele et al., 2019)

For men from working-class backgrounds intellectual work is often viewed as feminised, whilst physical work is seen as masculine and enables them to display strength and toughness (Fine et al., 1997). Those who worked in 'blue collar' jobs often referred to the dominance of masculinity in the working environment with strength prized and 'banter' common. Some masculinity that was lost due to being unable to keep up with physical tasks could be regained through being in leadership or managerial roles with work delegated downwards. However, this had to be carefully managed to maintain the respect of their workforce. Roger describes putting on a front to appear confident and avoid showing weakness, whilst Travis adopts bravado as a protective strategy enabling him to centre his masculinity around taking responsibility for his health:

> *I'm half the man I was. That's not nice … it's a front I have to put up, erm, it's a real front because, you know, if people think you are weak they'll take advantage of you. (Roger, 55yrs, Parkinson's disease, UK)* (Gibson & Kierans, 2017)

Travis *Testosterone just flows through the job site, it's kind of a joke really but nowadays […] I think of my health more today than I ever have, 'cause it really gets, it really got serious, you know, I want to stick around [laughs], so you drill that hole, you climb and get that ladder, I don't care what you think of me, whatever ….*

CF *So is, is there the thought that people might think badly of you for not being able to …*

Travis *Well I don't, like I said before guys want to be strong and support themselves, you know, so when you can't do that it's, it plays on you a little bit. (43yrs, systemic sclerosis, White American)*

In both physical jobs and desk jobs, when men were unable to perform their work to the standard that they held themselves to then they were often left feeling embarrassed or frustrated:

Mark *Myself, obviously with the type of job I do, I have to get other people now to lift heavy things, or where I used to lift a heavy boiler off the wall, I can't do it anymore, it's impossible.*

Paul *No, I had a nice shop, good sales, good footfall, fishing tackle, in the end I had to tell the customers, 'Yes sir, that's £44.99, could you bring it to the counter?' because I couldn't pick it up.*

Tom *You feel such a plonker.*
(Focus group of men with rheumatoid arthritis, UK)

> *I am frustrated that I have no stamina, that I'm such a weakling. That I can't just suck it up and then stay at work, and that I have to go home early. (Janus, 23yrs ankylosing spondylitis, Danish)* (Primholdt et al., 2017)

The value of working life for men was not only in protecting their masculine status as the provider and/or demonstrating strength and competence. Men's social support often comes in the form of engaging in shared tasks when they work side by side, and stand (literally or metaphorically) shoulder to shoulder. Thus, for many men their social networks were entrenched in their working life, and they were often reluctant to relinquish this:

> *Erm, I spoke to my bank manager. I won't say I'm loaded, but I've got some money in the bank, and he says, 'you've got enough to keep you going until you retire, then you go onto your pension, get all your pensions'. But … I do enjoy working, I mean, I enjoy being with the lads and everything else. It's all … all fellows, I'm with, no women. (Will, 61yrs, rheumatoid arthritis, White British)*

2.5 The Man of the House

Men with long-term conditions discussed the broader impact on their role in the home and within the family. In interviews with men with prostate cancer, Prof. John Oliffe asked men, *"When do you most feel like a man?"*, and many of the responses were related to traditional masculine protector and provider roles:

> *I pride myself as a bit of a handyman ... so lumping wood around and hammers and saws ... when I'm with my granddaughter. ... I still fill the old function footing the bill for bloody near everything. ... I'm able to be a good provider. (Kevin, advanced prostate cancer, Australian)* (Oliffe, 2006)

Engaging in DIY or other manual home improvement tasks can play a role in the construction of domestic masculinity. For those in non-physical or 'intellectual' jobs (as previously discussed often perceived by those from working-class backgrounds as more 'feminised') these manual domestic roles can provide a way for men to align themselves with a form of masculinity based on strength and physical prowess. Engaging in craftsman-like manual labour can be a form of 'therapeutic class tourism', which can provide men with a sense of superiority over other men within their work and social environments. In contrast, for men from working-class backgrounds, performing manual tasks within the home often enables them to demonstrate physical prowess and fulfil a protector and provider role in the family, which may be even more important if they are unable to fulfil the role of breadwinner due to illness (Moisio et al., 2013). Thus, for men across the social classes losing the ability to perform these manual tasks in the home due to illness could be experienced as losing 'man points' (De Visser & McDonnell, 2013).

Men throughout the literature and my own studies mentioned feeling the loss of being able to fulfil manual roles in the home. Often 'banter' was used to express this amongst other men within the focus group environment:

> *But, you know, as a man, yes, I suppose you always feel that as a man you should be the main person doing the lawns, the gardens, round the house, et cetera, et cetera, and sometimes it's frustrating when I'm sitting there in the garden watching the wife do it. I think not. [laughter]. (Mike, 60yrs, rheumatoid arthritis, White British)*

In the role of husband or partner many men (both straight and gay) cited their spouses or partners as a key source of support, but also the person who was most impacted by their illness. This could be through picking up the slack with tasks in the home, missing out on things they used to do as a couple that the men were no longer able to do, taking on a care-giver role, or sharing in the worries about the men's health. Many men acknowledged this impact on their partners, and some worried about the future of their relationship:

[M]y best would have been my partner … it's a lonely place being a gay man without support like that, especially if you don't have a partner. (Kevin, 47yrs, prostate cancer, Irish) (McConkey & Holborn, 2018)

I almost feel guilty, like I've stolen something from her by me being ill. I worry then that she will stop loving me. (Paul, 42yrs, chronic fatigue syndrome, White British) (Snell et al., 2023)

For those men who were fathers, being unable to play with their children in the way they wanted to was described as *"the worst part of this disease"* (man with ankylosing spondylitis) (Avrech Bar et al., 2021). Whilst in the past fatherhood was traditionally seen as a more hands-off role with nurturing and child-rearing seen as the women's domain, modern constructions of 'good' fatherhood reject an emotional lack of availability and praise hands-on involvement. To meet these expectations of an active father role whilst retaining masculine status, paternal care is often distinguished from maternal care through drawing on masculine traits such as toughness, athleticism, and autonomy (Randles, 2018). Thus, many of the men talked about the loss of the ability to engage in physical play with their children. Both Emil and Steve's accounts describe feeling as though they've lost esteem in their children's eyes, no longer seen as the invincible superhero. Both men describe pushing their bodies to their limits, and planning their symptom management in an effort to fulfil what some versions of hegemonic masculinity dictate is the way a man should interact with their child:

My pride's hurting me because my kids used to look up to me. I used to put both my kids on my shoulders, go to the park for about three or four hours sometimes. I can't even lift them and they want to play with me, they want to do things and I have to force myself to do these things with them, and as soon as like they're done I literally can't even feel my body I'm so numb, and it's the most normal thing, like to kick a ball in the house, play Lego or something, but my body's so stiff I can't do anything. (Emil, 37yrs, systemic sclerosis, Black British)

I used to play fight with him [son] and everything, pick him up and chuck him up the garden and stuff like that and I just can't anymore. It's just like … it's just so frustrating, not so much for me, but for him because he's always been used to Dad being … sons look at dads as being just like, 'Dad, you're invincible,' and then all of sudden you can't do it. […] That's the biggest thing I suppose out of everything, I can put up with everything else, but when my boy turns around and says to me, 'Why can't you come and play football with me dad?' that really, really hurts. That's the one thing I … I almost want him to grow up, I almost want him to be seventeen or eighteen so he doesn't want Dad to play football with him anymore. […] I mean stupid things like playing on the X-Box […] I'm thinking how many steroid tablets am I going to need to take to be able to use the controller properly? (Steve, 44yrs, rheumatoid arthritis, White British)

Despite long-term conditions interfering with the ability to engage in active play, some men emphasise that this does not affect their ability to be good fathers. However, whilst able to acknowledge the value of emotional and intellectual support, they still struggle to reconcile the loss of being the 'play figure' in their child's life:

Just because you're physically disabled doesn't mean you're not going to be a good father […] always be there for your child, emotionally, supportive. I mean be there for advice, as a shoulder to cry on, and be there to share your triumphs too. I mean father is the play figure, too, right? And that's the biggest part I have struggling with this. How do I be that play figure, that big tumbly, wrestly dad? (Colin, 50yrs, psoriatic arthritis, Canadian) (Avrech Bar et al., 2021)

Whilst some grandfathers choose to engage in potentially risky embodiments of masculinity such as physical play, others emphasise their wisdom and experience (Tarrant, 2013). Thus, some men who had become grandfathers were affected by this loss of being able to engage in physical play with their grandchildren, whilst others were more pragmatic and embraced not having to worry about the responsibility if they didn't feel well enough. Some weren't well enough to interact with energetic grandchildren, and this is discussed in the below quote using humour and bravado. However, it is important to consider this in the context of research that suggests positive interactions between grandfathers and grandsons are related to fewer depressive symptoms and positive affect in older men (Bates & Taylor, 2012):

So, when the grandson comes here it's kind of erm, it's nice. But there's things I can't do with him that I'd like to. I can't pick him up. So I can play with him if he's sitting here or I can read to him or we can watch TV but I guess I can't sort of pick him up and throw him around like his dad does. (John, 61yrs, rheumatoid arthritis, White British) (Flurey et al., 2018b)

They've got their parents, I did what I had to do, I got to worry about me now. I don't care what they think, it's all on me now, and my wife come with me, and you'll come to grandma all you want, grandpa ain't got time for you [laughing]. (Jacob, 62yrs, systemic sclerosis, African American)

2.6 Summary

Long-term conditions can pose significant challenges to masculinity through limiting men's ability for self-reliance, independence, and reducing the ways in which they're able to enact power and control. Men's social interactions often take the form of participating in shared activities, so when men are no longer physically able to engage in these, they can begin to lose their social support networks. Men's self-worth and masculinity is often tied up in their occupational status, and they can feel real or implied pressure to fulfil a breadwinner role. This can cause men to prioritise paid work over their health and wellbeing. For those no longer able to work due to a long-term condition this can cause them to question their purpose and value with associated impact on their mental wellbeing. Thus, it can be important that clinicians encourage men to remain in paid work and support them to do so in a way that is safe for their disease management. Traditional masculine protector and provider roles within the family are also challenged by long-term conditions. For men who are fathers and grandfathers the loss of ability to engage in physical play with children is particularly difficult to come to terms with.

References

Alexis, O., & Worsley, A. J. (2018). A meta-synthesis of qualitative studies exploring men's sense of masculinity post-prostate cancer treatment. *Cancer Nursing, 41*(4), 298–310. https://doi.org/10.1097/NCC.0000000000000509

Avrech Bar, M., Dao, T. T., DeBlock Vlodarchyk, L. R., & Backman, C. L. (2021). Fatherhood experiences of men with inflammatory arthritis: A preliminary grounded theory. *Arthritis Care & Research, 73*(6), 885–892. https://doi.org/10.1002/ACR.24189

Bamidele, O., McGarvey, H., Lagan, B. M., Parahoo, K., Chinegwundoh, M. B. E., & F., & McCaughan, E. (2019). "Man in the driving seat": A grounded theory study of the psychosocial experiences of Black African and

Black Caribbean men treated for prostate cancer and their partners. *Psycho-Oncology, 28*(8), 1712–1720. https://doi.org/10.1002/PON.5150
Bates, J. S., & Taylor, A. C. (2012). Grandfather involvement and aging men's mental health. *American Journal of Men's Health, 6*(3), 229–239. https://doi.org/10.1177/1557988311430249
Bauer, G. (2016). Gender roles, comparative advantages and the life course: The division of domestic labor in same-sex and different-sex couples. *European Journal of Population, 32*(1), 99–128. https://doi.org/10.1007/S10680-015-9363-Z
Connell, R. W. (2005). *Masculinities* (2nd ed.). University of California Press.
De Visser, R. O., & McDonnell, E. J. (2013). "Man points": Masculine capital and young men's health. *Health Psychology, 32*(1), 5–14. https://doi.org/10.1037/A0029045
Donnelly, T. T., Suwaidi, J. M., Al-Qahtani, A., Asaad, N., & Singh, R. (2019). Arab men and women's conceptualization of mental health and depression: A qualitative study from the Middle East. *Journal of Immigrant and Minority Health, 21*(5), 1102–1114. https://doi.org/10.1007/S10903-018-0809-3
Fine, M., Weis, L., Addelston, J., & Marusza, J. (1997). (In)secure times: Constructing white working-class masculinities in the late 20th century. *Gender & Society, 11*(1), 52–68.
Flurey, C., Hewlett, S., Rodham, K., White, A., Noddings, R., & Kirwan, J. (2016b). "You obviously just have to put on a brave face": A qualitative study of the experiences and coping styles of men with rheumatoid arthritis. *Arthritis Care & Research, 69*(3), 330–337.
Flurey, C., Hewlett, S., Rodham, K., White, A., Noddings, R., & Kirwan, J. R. (2016c). Identifying different typologies of experiences and coping strategies in men with rheumatoid arthritis: A Q-methodology study. *BMJ Open, 6*(10), e012051. https://doi.org/10.1136/bmjopen-2016-012051
Flurey, C., Pauling, J. D., Saketkoo, L. A., Denton, C. P., Galdas, P., Khanna, D., Williams, A., & Hughes, M. (2022). 'I turned in my man card': A qualitative study of the experiences, coping styles and support needs of men with systemic sclerosis. *Rheumatology, 62*(6), 2160–2167. https://doi.org/10.1093/RHEUMATOLOGY/KEAC585
Flurey, C., White, A., Rodham, K., Kirwan, J., Noddings, R., & Hewlett, S. (2018b). 'Everyone assumes a man to be quite strong': Men, masculinity and rheumatoid arthritis: A case-study approach. *Sociology of Health & Illness, 40*(1), 115–129.
Gibson, G., & Kierans, C. (2017). Ageing, masculinity and Parkinson's disease: Embodied perspectives. *Sociology of Health & Illness, 39*(4), 532–546. https://doi.org/10.1111/1467-9566.12508

Jaspers, E., & Verbakel, E. (2013). The division of paid labor in same-sex couples in the Netherlands. *Sex Roles, 68*, 335–348. https://doi.org/10.1007/S11199-012-0235-2

Khazen, M. (2022). Power dynamics in doctor-patient relationships: A qualitative study examining how cultural and personal relationships facilitate medication requests in a minority with collectivist attributes. *Patient Education and Counselling, 105*(7), 2038–2044.

Lack, S., Noddings, R., & Hewlett, S. (2011). Men's experiences of rheumatoid arthritis: An inductive thematic analysis. *Musculoskeletal Care, 9*(2), 102–112. https://doi.org/10.1002/msc.203

Mazar, I., & Moorman, S. M. (2021). "I want that life a lot…how on earth do I get that?" Examining challenges for men with Barth Syndrome in their transitions to adulthood. *Journal of Patient Experience, 8*. https://doi.org/10.1177/23743735211060783

McConkey, R. W., & Holborn, C. (2018). Exploring the lived experience of gay men with prostate cancer: A phenomenological study. *European Journal of Oncology Nursing, 33*, 62–69. https://doi.org/10.1016/j.ejon.2018.01.013

Minns Lowe, C. J., Toye, F., & Barker, K. L. (2019). Men's experiences of having osteoporosis vertebral fractures: A qualitative study using interpretative phenomenological analyses. *Osteoporosis International, 30*(7), 1403–1412. https://doi.org/10.1007/S00198-019-04973-0

Moisio, R., Arnould, E., & Gentry, J. (2013). Productive consumption in the class-mediated construction of domestic masculinity: Do-it-yourself (DIY) home improvement in men's identity work. *Journal of Consumer Research, 40*(2), 298–316.

O'Brien, R., Hart, G. J., & Hunt, K. (2007). "Standing out from the herd": Men renegotiating masculinity in relation to their experience of illness. *International Journal of Men's Health, 6*(3), 178–200.

Oliffe, J. (2006). Embodied masculinity and androgen deprivation therapy. *Sociology of Health & Illness, 28*(4), 410–432. https://doi.org/10.1111/J.1467-9566.2006.00499.X

Primholdt, N., Primdahl, J., & Hendricks, O. (2017). A difficult diagnosis: A qualitative study of the daily lives of young men diagnosed with ankylosing spondylitis. *Musculoskeletal Care, 15*(2), 140–149. https://doi.org/10.1002/MSC.1155

Quincey, K., Williamson, I., & Wildbur, D. (2021). Men with breast cancer and their encounters with masculinity: An interpretative phenomenological analysis using photography. *Psychology of Men and Masculinity, 22*(4), 690–703. https://doi.org/10.1037/MEN0000344

Randles, J. (2018). "Manning up" to be a good father: Hybrid fatherhood, masculinity, and U.S. responsible fatherhood policy. *Gender and Society, 32*(4), 516–539. https://doi.org/10.1177/0891243218770364

Salifu, Y., Almack, K., & Caswell, G. (2023). 'Out of the frying pan into the fire': A qualitative study of the impact on masculinity for men living with advanced prostate cancer. *Palliative Care and Social Practice, 17.* https://doi.org/10.1177/26323524231176829/

Sallinen, M., Mengshoel, A. M., & Solbrække, K. N. (2019). "I can't have it; I am a man. A young man!"—men, fibromyalgia and masculinity in a Nordic context. *International Journal of Qualitative Studies on Health and Well-Being, 14*(1). https://doi.org/10.1080/17482631.2019.1676974

Schrock, D., & Schwalbe, M. (2009). Men, masculinity, and manhood acts. *Annual Review of Sociology, 35*, 277–295.

Snell, G. E., Seage, C. H., & Mercer, J. (2023). A phenomenological study on the lived experience of men with chronic fatigue syndrome. *Journal of Health Psychology.* https://doi.org/10.1177/13591053231186385

Stapleton, S., & Pattison, N. (2014). The lived experience of men with advanced cancer in relation to their perceptions of masculinity: A qualitative phenomenological study. *Journal of Clinical Nursing, 24*(7–8), 1069–1078. https://doi.org/10.1111/jocn.12713

Tarrant, A. (2013). Grandfathering as spatio-temporal practice: Conceptualizing performances of ageing masculinities in contemporary familial carescapes. *Social & Cultural Geography, 14*(2), 192–210.

Vigorito, A. J., & Curry, T. J. (1998). Marketing masculinity: Gender identity and popular magazines. *Sex Roles, 39*(1–2), 135–152.

Warner, L. R., & Shields, S. A. (2007). The perception of crying in women and men: Angry tears, sad tears, and the "right way" to cry. In U. Hess & P. Philippot (Eds.), *Group dynamics and emotional expression* (pp. 92–117). Cambridge University Press.

CHAPTER 3

Mental Wellbeing

"I was in tears on the garage floor"

The focus of this book is on physical long-term conditions, but as we've established in the previous chapter the impact of a physical condition can affect men's identity, self-esteem, and self-worth, all of which can affect their mental health and wellbeing. In rheumatoid arthritis, depression and anxiety have been shown to be associated with poorer physical health outcomes and treatment response (Matcham et al., 2015). Thus, if men with long-term conditions are struggling with mental wellbeing, this may also affect their physical symptom management and clinical outcomes.

It is beyond the scope of this book to include mental health conditions throughout. However, there is much that can be learnt from the mental health literature about the way men discuss and cope with psychological distress to inform our understanding of this in the context of living with a physical long-term condition. Thus, this chapter will draw from the literature on mental health conditions such as anxiety and depression to improve our understanding of men's mental wellbeing.

3.1 Mental Health and Gender

In the general population, the prevalence of depression is lower in men than women, yet men have higher rates of suicide than women (OECD, 2017). The reasons for this paradox are likely multifaceted. For example,

C. Flurey, *Talking Men's Health*,
https://doi.org/10.1007/978-3-031-62593-0_3

men are more likely to choose more lethal forms of suicide, with men being more likely (75%) to complete suicide, and women being slightly more likely (57%) to attempt suicide (Mergl et al., 2015). However, we are also less likely to recognise the way men express psychological distress and some healthcare professionals may be less comfortable in addressing male distress, which could discourage disclosure. Men tend to be less likely to raise psychological issues themselves (Ridge et al., 2011), and depression in men often seems to be hidden in antisocial and risk-taking behaviours (e.g., drug and alcohol abuse, self-harm, suicide, road rage, sexual risk-taking, gambling, aggression, and violence) (Brownhill et al., 2005). Commonly utilised measures for depression are less sensitive in men than women. The Gotland Male Depression Scale—specifically developed to identify depression in men—has been shown to be significantly more effective at recognising men's distress than traditional clinical measures (Sigurdsson et al., 2015; Zierau et al., 2002).

Men with long-term conditions may be at greater risk of mental health issues than the general population of men. For example, primary care patients with vertebral fractures have been found to be at increased risk of self-harm compared to matched patients without fractures. Male patients with vertebral fractures showed the greatest risk of self-harm across study participants. These men had four times the levels of self-harm behaviours compared to men who were the same age and characteristics as them but without fractures. This contrasts with higher rates of self-harm for women seen in the general population, which the authors suggested may be explained in part by the impact on masculinity of being diagnosed with an 'old women's disease'. However, it should also be noted that men with increased fracture risk did also often have underlying causes such as medication use (steroids), hormone-related conditions (e.g., hypogonadism), or lifestyle behaviours (e.g., smoking), which can all be associated with higher instances of self-harm and mental illness diagnosis (Prior et al., 2021).

Gender doesn't exist in a vacuum, and wider determinants of health also contribute to the impact on mental health. Race-based everyday discrimination is significantly associated with suicide ideation (Goodwill et al., 2019), and victimisation and discrimination is associated with depression, suicide ideation, alcohol misuse, suicide attempt history, and self-harm in people with LGBTQ identities (Busby et al., 2020). Everyday forms of discrimination, referred to as "micro-aggressions" (such as, You speak English quite well!"), have the potential to be more stressful than overt acts of racism because they are repetitive and subtle (Hankerson et al., 2015). Clinician bias can also contribute to missed or incorrect diagnosis, with negative perceptions of Black men affecting diagnostic assessment. Underestimating Black men's intelligence can result in healthcare professionals minimising their mental health issues. Further, misinterpreting cultural mistrust of healthcare professionals with pathological symptoms has led to more African American men being diagnosed with schizophrenia or other psychotic disorders than their White counterparts, who are more likely to be diagnosed with mood disorders (Hankerson et al., 2015).

Thus, it is important to highlight that men from marginalised groups may be at additional risk of depression or depressive symptoms, with additional institutional barriers to receiving a diagnosis. Clinicians should be conscious of the way they interact with people from marginalised groups and work to recognise their unconscious biases to avoid perpetuating negative and discriminatory experiences of care. Cultural mistrust of healthcare professionals and the impact of this on help-seeking behaviours will be discussed further in Chap. 8.

3.2 Challenges to Mental Wellbeing

As we've seen in the previous chapter, the limitations imposed by living with a long-term condition can challenge masculine ideals such as strength, stoicism, and self-reliance, which in turn can challenge men's sense of value and self-worth. Will (below) describes this psychological impact that a loss of control and increased reliance on others can have. He explains how this is coupled with low mood from persistent pain. He goes on to describe a potentially vicious cycle of pain causing low mood, leading to a lack of motivation to engage in self-management behaviours, which in turn further exacerbates pain:

> *Er, psychologically I think it was a bit of a problem because it puts you in a position where you have to ask for help and it's not a very sort of macho thing. Sort of most … we're sort of brought up to be like in charge of things and doing things for other people, rather than having to ask them to do things for us. So that took a fair bit of mental adjustment. And the pain as well, I mean, sometimes I get periods of anything up to 10 days when I'm bedridden, so that brings on depression as well, because you're in so much pain you can't do anything, so the depression makes it harder for you to get up even when the pain's gone a bit, but that means the pain gets worse again because you're not doing any exercise*

and that. So that's ... there are a few sort of psychological sort of kickbacks on it. (Will, 61yrs, rheumatoid arthritis, White British) (Flurey et al., 2016b)

This link between mental wellbeing and the impact of physical restrictions challenging men's value and self-worth aligns with findings that patients with cancer who feel demoralised (a sense of helplessness and incompetence, resulting in the feeling of lost significance and purpose) are significantly more likely to be depressed (Tang et al., 2015). This connection is explicitly made by a participant (below) from a study focusing on how Arab patients with cardiovascular disease conceptualise mental health and depression. The participant uses the word '*oppress*' indicating a strong sense of not only loss of control but that this control has been relinquished to others. This highlights the importance of supporting men with long-term conditions to find ways to still feel valuable and useful, and regain control:

Mental health problems occur when the person doesn't have a desire towards life. He feels that all people oppress him. He doesn't feel he has any value in the society. This for sure will isolate him from people completely [and causes mental illness]. (cardiovascular disease, Arabic) (Donnelly et al., 2019)

As discussed in Chap. 2 one important way that long-term conditions can affect masculinity is through the impact it can have on job roles and finances. Whether this is feeling less competent at a job, no longer being able to work, having hours or roles reduced, or the way they are treated by colleagues. Looking to the depression literature, job loss can be a trigger for men's depression, with being 'let go' or fired being particularly distressing. For many men retirement may not be a welcome end to their working life, but instead represents a loss of routine, and erosion of purpose (Oliffe et al., 2013). Additionally, as discussed in Chap. 2, loss of work for men may also result in the loss of a key social support structure.

A previous longitudinal study found that men with rheumatoid arthritis who were able to remain in paid work reported significantly lower levels of negative affect and somatic complaints than women with rheumatoid arthritis in paid work. However, men with rheumatoid arthritis who had stopped working reported significantly higher distress scores than women with rheumatoid arthritis who had stopped working. Only one-third of the variance in depressive symptoms could be accounted for by socioeconomic status, disease status, work demands, and work autonomy (Fifield et al., 1996). This indicates there is something specific to men linking paid work and their psychological outcomes, which highlights the importance of men remaining in work for their mental wellbeing.

Throughout my own studies and the long-term conditions literature, men discuss the impact of loss of work on their mental wellbeing. Frank (below) describes the mental health impact caused by the loss of value and purpose due to losing his job. He expresses the loss of not just the job itself but the lifestyle, identity, and self-worth that went with this. There is also the unfairness of losing a valued job due to the limitations imposed by rheumatoid arthritis to come to terms with. He explains this as so much harder to deal with than the physical impact of pain, making the comparison to a physical injury that can be recovered from. We will revisit Frank later in this chapter (Sect. 3.6) and look at how he eventually spoke to the medical team about his mental health:

> *But you know what it's like playing rugby, you get hurt and it hurts doesn't it? You break bones and you're playing again in three weeks aren't you, you break your nose you play in the next week. But you get used to that, the pain is one thing but I think … I don't know. But I think it was because I could see no way forward in life. I got laid off from the job I loved, I absolutely adored the job […] and all of a sudden they says goodbye. You just think well get going like. I sat at home on the Monday morning and I thought to myself what do I do? What do I do? Been a busy man all my life and all of a sudden wallop you're gone. Working seven days a week, 12 hours a day and all this and it was wonderful, wonderful lifestyle but all of a sudden you're locked in your house, doors closed and you're finished Mr. And it tore me apart, it really did and that went on for about, I don't know, six months before I got dragged down the doctors like. I was pretty well literally dragged too. (Frank, 75yrs, rheumatoid arthritis, White British)*

The following quote illustrates the extent of the mental health impact that job loss can have on men. The loss of the breadwinner role may have a particularly marked impact in cultures with more defined gender roles, which may provoke feelings of shame and impact their status in society:

> *[…] in the past, I had thought of ending my life when things were tough. I've suffered. I have. For a man like me to have no cedi (unit of Ghanaian currency) on me, it is a sad story [Tears dropping, interview paused as participant showed emotion in the interview]. (Kwaku, prostate cancer, Ghanaian)* (Salifu et al., 2023)

In addition to the impact of their condition on abilities and roles, it is also worth mentioning that some men experienced an impact on their mental wellbeing due to medication side effects. Men receiving androgen deprivation therapy for prostate cancer explained that they experienced mood swings and outbursts of anger that they had to learn to control:

> *I've found that I've got massively enraged in a spontaneous way. Something triggered it and it's like a step function. My temperament, all of a sudden there's this almighty change. I wanted to hit someone. At another time, I wanted to choke someone to death. I just controlled it and it subsided. (Archie, advanced prostate cancer, Anglo-Australian)* (Oliffe, 2006)

3.3 Talking About Mental Wellbeing

Throughout my studies men seemed to approach discussion about mental wellbeing with caution. When I directly asked about this in the focus group setting some men described their mental wellbeing in terms that emphasised strength and control: "*You've got to be mentally strong*" (David, rheumatoid arthritis). The quote from Mark (below) provides an example of this language and demonstrates how some men (whether consciously or unconsciously) actively distanced themselves from men who experience depression or low mood. Mark's use of the word 'fight' may be an attempt to frame what he seems to be (perhaps unintentionally) describing as a feminine issue in masculine terms:

> *I'm strong minded and I think you can get depression over it. I think most males will try and fight the depression, they will, within reason. To be honest I'm running a business, and I haven't got a choice. (Mark, 49yrs, rheumatoid arthritis, White British)*

Whilst these men often spoke sympathetically about other men who experienced low mood or depression, they were keen to emphasise that this wasn't their own experience. This may in part be a result of a certain amount of stigma that still surrounds mental health. Despite societal attitudes softening there is still a perception that depression can be overcome by 'mind over matter' with the implication that 'succumbing' to depression is a form of weakness. Men with depression in the literature discuss their symptoms not being taken seriously by others:

> *I've often heard people say 'Get a grip! Don't make such a fuss'. (Luke, 55–59yrs, depression, Germany)* (Staiger et al., 2020)

Whilst stigma surrounding mental health can be a barrier to men from all communities, research suggests it may be a particular issue for Black men's experience of mental health in comparison to other ethnic groups ("*not only in the general populace is there a stigma, but it's there in our community on a very strong level*" (Campbell & Mowbray, 2016)). Lack of education is often blamed for this, but this is likely a reductionist view that ignores the social and cultural context. In fact, stigmatising views often prevail and sometimes even strengthen following educational interventions (Rao et al., 2007). The precarious social status of Black men in Western countries might contribute to stronger stigmatising attitudes and behaviours towards mental health in Black communities. Mental illness or associating with people with mental illness can be viewed as a threat to social status or can challenge racial identity ("*crazy like those White people*" (Campbell & Mowbray, 2016)). This stigma within their own communities can create additional barriers for Black men to discuss or disclose mental health issues:

> *All they're gonna do is give me some medication and people are going to tease me. (Richard, 43yrs, depression, African American)* (Campbell & Mowbray, 2016)

Previous focus groups with men across a range of life experiences found they spoke more readily about physical illnesses (coronary heart disease and prostate cancer) than mental illness, with participants who had experienced depression being reluctant to define themselves as ill (O'Brien et al., 2007). However, when men did talk about experiencing mental wellbeing issues, language seemed important in framing this. Men were more likely to talk about being 'annoyed', 'frustrated', or 'stressed' rather than using words that directly indicated low mood. Some men relied on the biomedical model to frame depression in their explanations. This may serve to remove any self-blame, and reassure or remind themselves that there is a medical cause—they haven't 'failed' to be 'mentally strong' (Hoffman & Addis, 2021):

Erm, a feeling of slight depression I suppose, I, I am a medic so, I'm talking about depression in the medical sense. (Henry, 78yrs, systemic sclerosis, White British)

It is my brain. It is my chemistry. It is me. (male depression blogger) (Clarke & Van Amerom, 2008)

3.4 Men Don't Cry, Or Do They?

According to The Cure, "Boys don't cry" but of course that's not true. However, for many men there is still a social pressure to 'man up' and hide their emotions. Many of the men in my interviews and focus groups did speak openly about crying. This was often phrased as being driven to tears through frustration, which may be interpreted as a more 'manly' reason for feeling emotional:

I was in tears on the garage floor, because I'd got a drill and I couldn't get up off the floor. (David, 58yrs, rheumatoid arthritis, White British)

Crying is assumed to violate masculine norms regarding the importance of emotional control (Wong & Rochlen, 2005). There is a generation shift to some extent with younger men being more accepting of emotional expression in other men ("*It certainly is a generational thing: we're encouraged to be more open now*" (Fox, 2004)). However, when 2000 people were asked, 'When did you last cry?' men were far less likely (30%) than women (70%) to have cried (or perhaps more accurately to admit to crying) in the past month, with the same ratio across all age groups (from age 18 to 60+) (Fox, 2004). However, the expression of 'manly emotion' can be permissible (e.g., it is often acceptable for men to cry when their favourite football team loses) as it conveys a degree of self-control that remains consistent with hegemonic masculinity (Warner & Shields, 2007). This disclosure of crying in frustration can fit the description of 'manly emotion' as it relates to the experience of frustration with physical limitations that the majority of others in the focus group are likely to have experienced. In a focus group setting amongst other men, strength may also be found in taking the lead in discussing emotions. Whilst the above quote came from the focus group setting, interestingly in the follow-up interview setting, David was able to open up about emotions experienced due to more vulnerable feelings of helplessness:

> *You end up in tears because you just can't understand what's going on [...] that was why it was so downing because it come on so fast, you didn't know where it was going to stop. (David, 58yrs, rheumatoid arthritis, White British)*

Some men did feel able to more openly discuss their fears about the future in the focus groups. This seemed to happen when all or most other men in the group disclosed emotional impact, and the level of disclosure gradually increased to sharing and expressing vulnerabilities with each other:

> *For the first three months I used to cry every night, every night I used to cry. I used to go sit and cry and I told my partner, and she says, 'I, I'll sleep with you' [...] so I'm thinking, yeah, I want to look after my grandchildren, I want my grandchildren to remember me, you know, and, and all this goes through your mind. I still get that, every so often, maybe once a week, once a month, once every three months. You know, but and then I cry myself to sleep. (Karim, systemic sclerosis, British Asian)*

In some cultures, this expectation for men to uphold masculine bravery and resist crying is even more prevalent than others. In the below quote Keith particularly associates his identity as an African American man with the vulnerability felt when expressing emotion publicly. He describes this as a sign of weakness and compares himself to a prey animal. Situating this within a broader social context, it may be particularly important for Black men to present themselves as strong and invulnerable both to live up to masculine values within their own communities and to avoid being perceived as a victim making them a target for racially motivated aggression:

> *[F]or an African-American male to do that [cry] in public, you feel very vulnerable, you know? It's a sign of weakness. You know, it's like an Achilles heel. And especially if you came up in the streets, that's something you never want to do because, you know, it's like that little triple wildebeest: you don't stand a chance. [laughs] (Keith, 55yrs, African American, depression)* (Campbell & Mowbray, 2016)

In the Ghanaian language, 'barima ɛnsu' is a common expression meaning 'men don't cry'. One participant with prostate cancer resisted revealing his emotions in an initial interview to uphold these cultural beliefs, but shed tears and opened up in a subsequent interview demonstrating the importance of building rapport to support men to open up (Salifu et al., 2023):

> *I couldn't tell anyone about it. And no one asks me how I feel emotionally. But speaking to you the other time [during the first interview] and now, I felt I should share this with you and let off some 'steam'. (Kwaku, prostate cancer, Ghanaian)* (Salifu et al., 2023)

3.5 Wearing the Mask of Masculinity

In my own qualitative research and much of the literature it's apparent that although they may be initially cautious, men will talk about low mood or depression in the research setting. This challenges societal assumptions that men will be strong and silent in the face of vulnerability. In a focus group setting this may be helped by shared experiences with other men, providing validation for their experiences. Some men with depression have previously expressed a preference for speaking to 'a stranger' to avoid having to reveal a perceived weakness to someone they know due to pride or fear of the impact on their relationship (Emslie et al., 2007). Thus, although findings in this chapter challenge assumptions around men's unwillingness to talk there may still be a reluctance when it comes to disclosing issues related to mental wellbeing to friends and family. For some men, mental health wasn't seen as something men were 'supposed' to talk to each other about with some worrying about how breaking these social norms and expressing this vulnerability would affect their social status. This held men back from sharing with peer groups, or they carefully negotiated and navigated the level and nature of emotional expression they shared:

> *You're not supposed to open up to other guys about that. You're supposed to seem confident and strong and you can accomplish things on your own and stuff like that. … That's what proves your value to other people I think and so, by discussing it with other people … it just lowers your value … so you just shouldn't talk about it. (24yrs, depression, Canada)* (Tang et al., 2014)

> *There's always a limit to what you talk about. There's never a full-blown conversation about feelings and emotions but there always is in some sort of form … you can speak openly more to some than others. (Henry, 25yrs, anxiety, Welsh)* (Gough et al., 2021)

Both men and women can experience difficulty in finding the words to express mental health issues (Emslie et al., 2007). Men explained that physical injuries (e.g., football injuries) could be easier to talk about as "*people talk about those kind of things all the time*" (O'Brien et al., 2007). It may also be that physical injuries can be a mark of masculinity due to being injured through engaging in a masculine pursuit (e.g., sport, DIY). The social stigma that mental illness is something that can be overcome with enough 'mental strength' also means that physical impact is more easily understood than depression. Thus, men can find it easier to disclose physical rather than mental illness, or use physical impact to mask emotional impact:

> *It was easier to tell them at work that no, I couldn't drive because I had a sore back because my vertebrae [had been] broken than it was to say, "I feel really shitty today. I want a day off." It was much easier to say, "My back's killing me. I'm not coming in." That's a physical versus a mental thing. (55yrs, depression, Canada)* (Oliffe et al., 2013)

This is important to remember when considering speaking to men in the clinical environment, where for long-term conditions physical impact is often the focus of consultations. Although healthcare professionals may ask indirectly about mental wellbeing (e.g., how are you doing today), for many men unless they are asked explicitly about mental wellbeing, they may be unlikely to raise this themselves (see Sect. 3.8 for suggestions of how to ask men about mental wellbeing based on the work of the charity Talk Club):

> *I think they probably ask how, well they ask how I've been and how I am being, I mean I tend to take that from an RA [rheumatoid arthritis] perspective rather than an overall perspective. Erm, whether that's right or not I don't know. I mean I don't know whether they mean it as a general health thing or just from an RA perspective. I don't really know. I don't know they ever split the question. (John, 61yrs, rheumatoid arthritis, White British)*

With concerns about the stigma of depression, many men discuss making attempts to mask their low mood. Some do this by withdrawing from others, and as the quote below demonstrates some force themselves to put on a front. This is an important reminder that we may never know how much someone is struggling unless we ask:

I'll feel really bad sometimes, and I don't want to shave. And I don't want to do, and it's like, but I do it anyway, 'cause I don't want anybody to know. So I clean up and I shave and I get tight and I go out in the world, and no one knows. (depression, USA) (Rochlen et al., 2010)

For many men their spouses and partners are their main source of support. However, as I will discuss in Chap. 7, some men mask the full impact of their condition from those closest to them due to concerns about 'burdening' them or adding to their worries. This could also be true of emotional impact, which was often less likely to be discussed with their families than physical impact:

CF *And is that something you're able to talk to other people about, the low mood, do you talk to your wives?*
WADE *No, I keep that to myself.*
LIAM *I always keep that on the down low.*
(Focus group with men with systemic sclerosis, USA)

3.6 Role of Family

Whilst men may not always find it easy to discuss emotional issues with those closest to them, for many men with depression their family were a key source of support. Family can provide emotional support and encouragement, promote depression management in the home, and facilitate communication about depression at primary care visits (Hinton et al., 2015):

Then my kid, she picked my spirits back up again. You know, hollering at me, 'you dummy, you are worth more than what you say you are'. Because all of my life, my old man told me that I wasn't worth shit. I was worthless. (depression, American) (Hinton et al., 2015)

For men with depression, disclosure to a friend or partner could make them feel less vulnerable than speaking to a healthcare professional (Johnson et al., 2012). As with men with physical long-term conditions, married or partnered men with depression often seemed to cope as a team with their partner describing support with medication regimes and arranging appointments:

> *My wife is the pillar of my strength. She labels all of my medicines. She organizes how to take them, how many time, I mean how many milligrams. … So she is the driving force as far as my medical support. (depression, USA)* (Hinton et al., 2015)

Single or closeted gay men tend to report lower levels of emotional support and have described a lonely experience of long-term conditions (McConkey & Holborn, 2018). Emotional support for men's depression within gay relationships comes with potential additional complexities of a male partner having their own masculinity values to live up to. However, research suggests gay men may offer support to their depressed partners with little reference to gender roles:

> *I just saw it as something that I needed to do, it was kind of my role to take care of him. … I saw that I needed to protect him and take care of him and that kind of thing. (gay partner of depressed man, USA)* (Thomeer et al., 2015)

Family can play a key role in encouraging men to seek help for low mood or depression, which the following excerpt from Frank demonstrates well. Frank was experiencing depression resulting from losing his job following his diagnosis. When he went for his clinical appointment, he wasn't explicitly asked about emotional issues and so focused on his physical symptoms. He explains that if his adult son hadn't insisted that he went back to the doctor then "*I don't know what would have happened*":

> *I was in tears at home, I wouldn't speak to anybody, I was snappy with my son, which is most unusual because we're best friends like. And he came in from work one day and he said, 'now listen you, sit down', I said 'I don't want to sit down'. He said, 'alright then', he said 'if you don't get down the doctors, I'm getting her up here'. I said, 'I'll think about it', he said 'no you won't get in the car I'll take you now', and he's a big lump, my son, he is a big lad, big, strong man. I said, 'okay then', so we went down […] if I hadn't of gone down there I don't know what would have happened, I wouldn't answer the phone, I wouldn't even answer the door. Just walking around the house, wouldn't go to the pub, nothing. (Frank, 75yrs, rheumatoid arthritis, White British)*

However, whilst family have the ability to provide much support and reassurance for men's mental wellbeing, they also have the power to trigger or worsen depression. The opinions and values of family can have a big impact, meaning that stigmatising views of depression, discouraging treatment, or undermining men's experiences can hinder their care:

> *Oh, those around [family] say, 'don't take that [anti-depressant], that's for locos [crazies]', this and that. (depression, Mexican)* (Hinton et al., 2015)

Family (often partner/spouse, parents, or adult children) can help with clinical appointments by bringing up issues men may be reluctant to disclose themselves. However, their presence can also hinder men feeling able to discuss certain issues that they may be trying to protect their family members from (such as mortality, see Chap. 6). Additionally, when men do open up to their families it is important to ensure they feel listened to, as moving into an amateur therapist role where men may feel 'analysed' can discourage emotional expression:

> *I can say to her, I'm really fed up and she says, sit down and we'll talk about it. There comes a point when she looks at me and she knows we have to talk. After the kids have gone to school I might start talking. Then she takes over, she tells me why I feel the way I do. Then I shut up. (depression, UK)* (Alexander, 2001)

3.7 Losing and Regaining Control

When men are no longer able to control their emotional distress, they become more likely to engage in ways that may be internally or externally destructive. This can mean engaging in risky, dangerous, or life threatening behaviours, or becoming angry, aggressive, or violent (Brownhill et al., 2005):

> *Just hit something, break anything ... you break things ... smash something, smash bottles ... yeah, just release some anger ... you just lash out real bad. (male student discussion on 'being down in the dumps', Australia)* (Brownhill et al., 2005)

This 'big build' of emotion may even lead to blaming others, self-harm, or suicidal behaviours (Brownhill et al., 2005). For example, men with penile cancer discussed how life was essentially focused on survival day by day. They expressed fears of cancer recurrence and suicidal ideation was experienced as a way of regaining control over an unpredictable future (Törnävä et al., 2022).

Whilst internally destructive behaviours seemed more commonly spoken about, some men did also discuss dealing with distress through taking it out on others. Some men expressed anger and frustration towards a medical system they felt was failing them (Alexis & Worsley, 2018). Others described becoming angry and aggressive towards loved ones, or in more extreme cases this behaviour carried into the workplace:

> *I flew off the handle 'cause I couldn't do it. I can't help it—I just get so irritable. I know I can do it, but I can't, you know? (Patient K, 61yrs, rheumatoid arthritis, UK)* (Lack et al., 2011)

> *They retired me early because of my depression and my posttraumatic stress. I was having trouble with people at work, you know. I started threatening people and I hit a student one time for being lippy. (66yrs, depression, Canada)* (Oliffe et al., 2013)

To re-establish control and cope with depression, men have emphasised the importance of moving from dependence to independence. This can be through taking control of their healthcare, reducing dependency on drugs, or even taking a form of comfort in knowing that suicide was an option they were currently choosing not to take (Emslie et al., 2006):

> *But at least to have control over whether you kill yourself or not, it's sort of the last thing that you've got control over. (DP05, 33yrs, bipolar depression, UK)* (Emslie et al., 2006)

Chapter 7 will discuss the various ways men with long-term conditions work to regain control of their lives through self-management.

3.8 'What's Your Number?': Encouraging Men to Talk About 'Mental Fitness'

Despite common social narratives that men don't open up we can see that given a safe, private, and trusted environment (see Chap. 9 for what contributes to this) men will attend groups for support with depression and anxiety (Cramer et al., 2014).

An exemplar format for engaging men in discussion about their mental health comes from Talk Club (Talk Club, 2024). Talk Club are a charity that brand themselves as 'a male mental fitness movement', harnessing masculine language to normalise taking care of mental health in the same way men may take care of their physical health through going to the gym. This aligns well with language previously discussed with men emphasising the importance of being 'mentally strong'.

Talk Club use a talking group format, which has the same structure each week providing a clear expectation of what will happen when men attend. Each group starts with asking everyone: "How are you? Out of 10?" (with 1 being 'rock bottom' and 10 being 'top of the world'). They find that putting a number on their feelings then helps men explain why they've chosen that number. Each man has a chance to speak without interruption, and they are not encouraged to engage in 'fixing' each other's 'problems'. At the end of each session men are then asked for their number again and anecdotally these numbers tend to increase through the positive effect of talking to the group, which reinforces the benefits of attending. Building on the idea that men often provide effective support whilst engaged in a shared activity (see Chap. 9), Talk Club have also broadened their remit out to include talk and exercise (e.g., talk and walk, talk and golf, talk and football). Acknowledging that men scoring at various points on their scale may have different needs, Talk Club have also expanded to include therapy groups (up to six men per group led by a qualified therapist) and will soon also offer one-to-one therapy. This allows them to provide appropriately staged support to men from zero to ten, enabling men to engage in 'mental fitness' at the right time for them and encourages accessing support long before hitting 'rock bottom'.

Talk Club's approach not only provides a useful format in considering developing support for mental wellbeing for men with long-term conditions, but their 1 to 10 scale is easy to adapt to promote discussion in clinical practice. The use of a number rather than language to facilitate conversation could be easily widely adopted. This also aligns with the use of numerical rating scales and visual analogue scales that are often used in clinical practice (e.g., for pain, or fatigue). In a Talk Club group this scale is used in the context of mental fitness, so "how are you? out of 10?" or "what's your number?" doesn't need any clarification here. In a clinical setting, it would be helpful to preface this with "in relation to your mental fitness" to avoid issues mentioned above of men with long-term conditions assuming healthcare professionals are only concerned with their physical health.

Once men are familiar with this scale, it may be much easier to tell you they are a one or two today than to verbalise "I'm struggling" or "I'm at rock bottom". Talk Club's "how are you? out of 10?" or "what's your number?" has the power to open the door for potentially much-needed conversations that could be missed by asking a more generic "how are you feeling?". Other examples of groups that work well to support men will be discussed in Chap. 9, which focuses on effective psychosocial support for men.

3.9 Summary

Depression and anxiety are associated with poorer physical health outcomes and response to treatment. Men with long-term conditions can experience challenges to their mental wellbeing through the various ways their condition impacts their lives and self-esteem. Despite popular narratives that men are reluctant to talk about emotional topics, they will often open up when given a safe, private, and trusted environment to do so. However, it may be important to men to emphasise aspects of their masculinity such as 'mental strength', and for some men stigma associated with mental illnesses may be navigated through emphasising biomedical causes of depression. Men from marginalised groups may be at greater risk of low mood or depression and may face greater barriers to seeking help and receiving appropriate care. Men are aware of social restrictions in emotional expression and may exert caution in who they will open up to and to what extent. Men's partners and family units can be an important source of support for mental wellbeing, and can be crucial in encouraging men to seek help for mental health issues such as depression. Asking men the simple question 'how are you? out of 10?' can be a safe and non-confrontational way of effectively opening up the conversation about mental wellbeing.

References

Alexander, J. (2001). Depressed men: An exploratory study of close relationships. *Journal of Psychiatric and Mental Health Nursing*, *8*(1), 67–75. https://doi.org/10.1111/j.1365-2850.2001.00354.x

Alexis, O., & Worsley, A. J. (2018). A meta-synthesis of qualitative studies exploring men's sense of masculinity post-prostate cancer treatment. *Cancer Nursing*, *41*(4), 298–310. https://doi.org/10.1097/NCC.0000000000000509

Brownhill, S., Wilhelm, K., Barclay, L., & Schmied, V. (2005). 'Big build': Hidden depression in men. *Australian and New Zealand Journal of Psychiatry, 39*(10), 921–931.

Busby, D. R., Horwitz, A. G., Zheng, K., Eisenberg, D., Harper, G. W., Albucher, R. C., Roberts, L. W., Coryell, W., Pistorello, J., & King, C. A. (2020). Suicide risk among gender and sexual minority college students: The roles of victimization, discrimination, connectedness, and identity affirmation. *Journal of Psychiatric Research, 121*, 182–188. https://doi.org/10.1016/J.JPSYCHIRES.2019.11.013

Campbell, R. D., & Mowbray, O. (2016). The stigma of depression: Black American experiences. *Journal of Ethnic and Cultural Diversity in Social Work, 25*(4), 253–269. https://doi.org/10.1080/15313204.2016.1187101

Clarke, J., & Van Amerom, G. (2008). A comparison of blogs by depressed men and women. *Issues in Mental Health Nursing, 29*(3), 243–264. https://doi.org/10.1080/01612840701869403

Cramer, H., Horwood, J., Payne, S., Araya, R., Lester, H., & Salisbury, C. (2014). Do depressed and anxious men do groups? What works and what are the barriers to help-seeking? *Primary Health Care Research & Development, 15*(3), 287–301.

Donnelly, T. T., Suwaidi, J. M., Al-Qahtani, A., Asaad, N., & Singh, R. (2019). Arab men and women's conceptualization of mental health and depression: A qualitative study from the Middle East. *Journal of Immigrant and Minority Health, 21*(5), 1102–1114. https://doi.org/10.1007/S10903-018-0809-3

Emslie, C., Ridge, D., Ziebland, S., & Hunt, K. (2006). Men's accounts of depression: Reconstructing or resisting hegemonic masculinity? *Social Science & Medicine, 62*(9), 2246–2257.

Emslie, C., Ridge, D., Ziebland, S., & Hunt, K. (2007). Exploring men's and women's experiences of depression and engagement with health professionals: More similarities than differences? A qualitative interview study. *BMC Family Practice, 8*(43). https://doi.org/10.1186/1471-2296-8-43

Fifield, J., Reisine, S., Sheehan, T. J., & McQuillan, J. (1996). Gender, paid work, and symptoms of emotional distress in rheumatoid arthritis patients. *Arthritis and Rheumatism, 39*(3), 427–435.

Flurey, C., Hewlett, S., Rodham, K., White, A., Noddings, R., & Kirwan, J. (2016b). "You obviously just have to put on a brave face": A qualitative study of the experiences and coping styles of men with rheumatoid arthritis. *Arthritis Care & Research, 69*(3), 330–337.

Fox, K. (2004). *The Kleenex® for men crying game report: A study of men and crying*. http://webmail.sirc.org/publik/crying_game.pdf

Goodwill, J., Taylor, R., & Watkins, D. (2019). Everyday discrimination, depressive symptoms, and suicide ideation among African American men. *Archives of*

Suicide Research, 25(1), 74–93. https://doi.org/10.1080/13811118.2019.1660287
Gough, B., Robertson, S., & Luck, H. (2021). Engendered expressions of anxiety: Men's emotional communications with women and other men. *Frontiers in Sociology, 6*. https://doi.org/10.3389/FSOC.2021.697356
Hankerson, S. H., Suite, D., & Bailey, R. K. (2015). Treatment disparities among African American men with depression: Implications for clinical practice. *Journal of Health Care for the Poor and Underserved, 26*(1), 21–34. https://doi.org/10.1353/hpu.2015.0012
Hinton, L., Apesoa-Varano, E. C., Unützer, J., Dwight-Johnson, M., Park, M., & Barker, J. C. (2015). A descriptive qualitative study of the roles of family members in older men's depression treatment from the perspectives of older men and primary care providers. *International Journal of Geriatric Psychiatry, 30*(5), 514–522. https://doi.org/10.1002/gps.4175
Hoffman, E., & Addis, M. (2021). Dilemmas of agency and blame in men's talk about depression. *Psychology of Men & Masculinities, 22*(4), 669–677.
Johnson, J. L., Oliffe, J. L., Kelly, M. T., Galdas, P., & Ogrodniczuk, J. S. (2012). Men's discourses of help-seeking in the context of depression. *Sociology of Health & Illness, 34*(3), 345–361. https://doi.org/10.1111/J.1467-9566.2011.01372.X
Lack, S., Noddings, R., & Hewlett, S. (2011). Men's experiences of rheumatoid arthritis: An inductive thematic analysis. *Musculoskeletal Care, 9*(2), 102–112. https://doi.org/10.1002/msc.203
Matcham, F., Norton, S., Scott, D. L., Steer, S., & Hotopf, M. (2015). Symptoms of depression and anxiety predict treatment response and long-term physical health outcomes in rheumatoid arthritis: Secondary analysis of a randomized controlled trial. *Rheumatology, 55*(2), 268–278.
McConkey, R. W., & Holborn, C. (2018). Exploring the lived experience of gay men with prostate cancer: A phenomenological study. *European Journal of Oncology Nursing, 33*, 62–69. https://doi.org/10.1016/j.ejon.2018.01.013
Mergl, R., Koburger, N., Heinrichs, K., Székely, A., Tóth, M. D., Coyne, J., Quintão, S., Arensman, E., Coffey, C., Maxwell, M., Värnik, A., Van Audenhove, C., McDaid, D., Sarchiapone, M., Schmidtke, A., Genz, A., Gusmão, R., & Hegerl, U. (2015). What are reasons for the large gender differences in the lethality of suicidal acts? An epidemiological analysis in four European countries. *PLoS ONE, 10*(7). https://doi.org/10.1371/JOURNAL.PONE.0129062
O'Brien, R., Hart, G. J., & Hunt, K. (2007). "Standing out from the herd": Men renegotiating masculinity in relation to their experience of illness. *International Journal of Men's Health, 6*(3), 178–200.
OECD. (2017). *Health at a glance 2017: OECD indicators.*

Oliffe, J. (2006). Embodied masculinity and androgen deprivation therapy. *Sociology of Health & Illness, 28*(4), 410–432. https://doi.org/10.1111/J.1467-9566.2006.00499.X
Oliffe, J. L., Rasmussen, B., Bottorff, J. L., Kelly, M. T., Galdas, P. M., Phinney, A., & Ogrodniczuk, J. S. (2013). Masculinities, work, and retirement among older men who experience depression. *Qualitative Health Research, 23*(12), 1626–1637. https://doi.org/10.1177/1049732313509408
Prior, J. A., Crawford-Manning, F., Whittle, R., Abdul-Sultan, A., Chew Graham, C. A., Muller, S., Shepherd, T. A., Sumathipala, A., Mallen, C. D., & Paskins, Z. (2021). Vertebral fracture as a risk factor for self-harm: A retrospective cohort study. *BMC Musculoskeletal Disorders, 22*(1). https://doi.org/10.1186/S12891-021-04631-9
Rao, D., Feinglass, J., & Corrigan, P. (2007). Racial and ethnic disparities in mental illness stigma. *Journal of Nervous and Mental Disease, 195*(12), 1020–1023. https://doi.org/10.1097/NMD.0b013e31815c046e
Ridge, D., Emslie, C., & White, A. (2011). Understanding how men experience, express and cope with mental distress: Where next? *Sociology of Health & Illness, 33*(1), 145–159.
Rochlen, A., Paterniti, D., Epstein, R., Duberstein, P., Willeford, L., & Kravitz, R. (2010). Barriers in diagnosing and treating men with depression: A focus group report. *American Journal of Men's Health, 4*(2), 167–175. https://doi.org/10.1177/1557988309335823
Salifu, Y., Almack, K., & Caswell, G. (2023). 'Out of the frying pan into the fire': A qualitative study of the impact on masculinity for men living with advanced prostate cancer. *Palliative Care and Social Practice, 17*. https://doi.org/10.1177/26323524231176829/
Sigurdsson, B., Palsson, S. P., Aevarsson, O., Olafsdottir, M., & Johannsson, M. (2015). Validity of Gotland Male Depression Scale for male depression in a community study: The Sudurnesjamenn study. *Journal of Affective Disorders, 173*, 81–89.
Staiger, T., Stiawa, M., Mueller-Stierlin, A. S., Kilian, R., Beschoner, P., Gündel, H., Becker, T., Frasch, K., Panzirsch, M., Schmauß, M., & Krumm, S. (2020). Masculinity and help-seeking among men with depression: A qualitative study. *Frontiers in Psychiatry, 11*. https://doi.org/10.3389/FPSYT.2020.599039
Talk Club. (2024). *Talk Club*. https://talkclub.org/
Tang, M., Oliffe, J., Galdas, P., Phinney, A., & Han, C. (2014). College men's depression-related help-seeking: A gender analysis. *Journal of Mental Health, 23*(5), 219–224. https://doi.org/10.3109/09638237.2014.910639
Tang, P. L., Wang, H. H., & Chou, F. H. (2015). A Systematic review and meta-analysis of demoralization and depression in patients with cancer. *Psychosomatics, 56*(6), 634–643. https://doi.org/10.1016/J.PSYM.2015.06.005
Thomeer, M. B., Reczek, C., & Umberson, D. (2015). Relationship dynamics around depression in gay and lesbian couples. *Social Science and Medicine, 147*, 38–46. https://doi.org/10.1016/j.socscimed.2015.10.048

Törnävä, M., Harju, E., Vasarainen, H., Pakarainen, T., Perttilä, I., & Kaipia, A. (2022). Men's experiences of the impact of penile cancer surgery on their lives: A qualitative study. *European Journal of Cancer Care, 31*(1), e13548. https://doi.org/10.1111/ECC.13548

Warner, L. R., & Shields, S. A. (2007). The perception of crying in women and men: Angry tears, sad tears, and the "right way" to cry. In U. Hess & P. Philippot (Eds.), *Group dynamics and emotional expression* (pp. 92–117). Cambridge University Press.

Wong, Y. J., & Rochlen, A. B. (2005). Demystifying men's emotional behavior: New directions and implications for counseling and research. *Psychology of Men & Masculinity, 6*, 62–72.

Zierau, F., Bille, A., Rutz, W., & Bech, P. (2002). The Gotland male depression scale: A validity study in patients with alcohol use disorder. *Nordic Journal of Psychiatry, 56*(4), 265–271.

CHAPTER 4

Self-image and Body Image

"I look in the mirror and think who's that?"

Body image is the term commonly used for the range of thoughts and feelings we have about our body. It includes the way we see our body (which may or may not represent how others see us), how we feel about our body, and how we think about our body. These thoughts and feelings can also affect the way we treat our bodies or our general behaviours. Self-image is the term for the overall way we see ourselves, which includes but is not limited to body image. Self-image is more broadly how we see, feel, and think about ourselves; how we think others see us; and whether these align with how we would like to be seen. Whilst this includes physical appearance, it can also include skills and attributes, values, and how we fit into societal norms or expectations. This chapter was initially planned to cover body image only, but there is so much overlap with this and men's self-image in relation to masculinity that I've chosen to present these concepts together.

4.1 Visible Differences

Social norms often dictate that appearance is the domain of women. Men should be effortlessly attractive without spending time or giving attention to their appearance. However, according to the Mental Health Foundation, 28% of men over 18 years have felt anxious due to body image issues

C. Flurey, *Talking Men's Health*,
https://doi.org/10.1007/978-3-031-62593-0_4

(Mental Health Foundation, 2023). Whilst societal understanding of men's body image issues is improving, it is still sufficiently unusual for male body image issues to be a topic of discussion that when soap operas run storylines relating to male eating disorders or body dysmorphia they trend on social media and receive media praise for raising awareness.

Patients with long-term conditions (whatever their gender) may be less likely to express concerns about their appearance to their medical team as there are often more pressing treatment priorities to consider. When combined with a social narrative that implies men shouldn't care about their appearance it may be even harder for men to raise these issues to their clinical team:

> *One of the things that I think's pretty unfair is that, because you're a man you shouldn't really care so much about your appearance. (Zahid, 41yrs, alopecia areata, UK)* (Zucchelli et al., 2022)

Systemic sclerosis can cause visible facial differences through rash-like discolouration, dry skin, and/or skin tightening around the mouth. When planning the topics I would cover in my systemic sclerosis focus groups with my clinician collaborators and patient research partner we chose to explicitly ask about the impact of these visible differences as this had not previously been addressed with men with systemic sclerosis. However, I was surprised to find that none of the men I spoke to were concerned with visible facial signs of systemic sclerosis. As Chris (below) notes, this may be something that would have been more of a concern when these men were younger (mean age of study participants: 58yrs). However, despite Chris saying he's not concerned about the appearance of dry skin on his face he still likens himself to a lizard. This comparison implies a feeling of unattractiveness, and he takes steps to resolve this through moisturising. Thus, his response may reflect adherence to generational social norms of men not caring about their appearance:

> *If I was in my 20s, I would be very conscious and upset by my face and my complexion and my skin, you know, trying to sort of shave this morning, sometimes it's much, much worse than this the dry skin situation, so that, it's like a blooming lizard by the time my skin's dried out and yes, I do use creams and all the rest of it but, you know, not now, not now, now I, you know, 55. (Chris, 55yrs, systemic sclerosis, White British)*

It is possible that due to the severity of systemic sclerosis, visible differences have become less important to these men. However, they were still concerned with bodily changes (e.g., weight and muscle loss), which I will discuss in Sect. 4.4. Despite these men's indifference, it is clear from the wider literature that many men with long-term conditions do experience a negative impact of changes to their appearance. In complete contrast to the men with systemic sclerosis from my focus groups, this Taiwanese man with oral cancer describes feelings of depression due to his altered appearance:

> *I felt very depressed and angry with my altered appearance, because I was totally unprepared; it was painful for me to accept this. The reason I felt depressed was that I saw myself slobbering … everyday … and that has affected my self-esteem. (oral cancer, Taiwanese)* (Hu et al., 2009)

It could be argued that the impact on this man is related more to the loss of function and control as he describes *'slobbering'* as the salient issue. However, other examples throughout the literature provide a more explicit discussion of the impact of altered appearance on men's body image and self-esteem. Men describe negative feelings towards their bodies due to visible differences. For example, Eammon describes his body with post-surgery scarring as ugly and feels unable to look at it:

> *I think it looks absolutely bloody awful so ugly looking … I can't stand in front of the mirror and look … I'll take off my shirt look around the room as I'm doing it then pull a t-shirt on … it's my perception because it's mine … I can't get over it. (Eammon, breast cancer, UK)* (Quincey et al., 2021)

Far from the narrative that men shouldn't care about their bodies, visible appearance differences can inhibit men from taking part in activities they used to enjoy. This may be a particular issue in fitness spaces where men's bodies are exposed. Here they may feel a heightened awareness of their bodies (and how they match up to a masculine ideal) in direct comparison to other male bodies, and can feel their bodies are being similarly assessed by others (Wagner, 2016):

> *I went to the gym regularly and did a lot of swimming. So my body appearance was on view (…) which slightly embarrassed me, you know the changes (…) probably because of my body image I didn't do any swimming for some time.*

> *(Henry, 74yrs, undergoing androgen deprivation therapy for prostate cancer, UK)* (Gentili et al., 2019)

Some men reclaimed the narrative and spoke in a way that embraced scarring from cancer surgery as a mark of heroism or survivorship. This was no longer a disfigured body causing shame or embarrassment. It is a body that was strong enough to withstand adversity and survive. This altered narrative enables men to align their altered body to masculine ideals of strength and bravery:

> *The surgery and my scar were going to tell a story. It is my battle wound. The scar is just going to be there, and it's a conversation piece. (P-16, breast cancer, USA)* (Potter et al., 2023)

4.2 Alopecia

The mixed views around how explicitly men discuss body image concerns continue into the literature surrounding alopecia (hair loss). Throughout the literature some men seemed to play down the impact of hair loss through comparing to women's experiences, highlighting the gendered importance of hair to women. Implicit in this comparison may be the societal expectation that as men they shouldn't be concerned about hair loss. Some men discussed practical frustrations with hair loss such as feeling the cold more but without acknowledging appearance concerns. One man who has lost his hair due to cancer treatment clearly emphasises the distinction between wearing a hat for functional rather than 'vanity' reasons:

> *I did wear a hat when I was out and about. That wasnae vanity, it was sensibility because I had nothing to protect my head so I wore my hat then. Other than that it didnae bother me. (P3, 63yrs, oropharyngeal cancer, Scottish)* (Rennie et al., 2018)

However, other men directly expressed distress at losing their hair. Men with alopecia areata compared this to men experiencing male pattern baldness, which they thought would be easier to accept. Male pattern baldness was described as '*sexualised*' (Zucchelli et al., 2022) due to the social narrative that bald men are more virile, with prominent bald masculine figures such as Bruce Willis and Terry Crews enhancing this perception. Whereas alopecia areata was described as setting them apart from other men due to patchy patterns of hair loss that isn't prominent in mainstream media. Zahid (below) expresses concerns about his hair loss patches marking him out as having a disease. Thus, there is perhaps more to body image concerns with men beyond simply the altered appearance. Through this altered appearance they are in danger of being seen as weakened due to illness, and of "*standing out form the herd*", distinct from other men (O'Brien et al., 2007):

> *The way that the hair goes [with AA] is not very pretty ... I think with male pattern baldness, it's more symmetrical and predictable ... it doesn't trigger other people's sense of 'Oh, there's disease here.' Whereas, with Alopecia Areata it looks like something is wrong. (Zahid, 41yrs, alopecia areata, UK)* (Zucchelli et al., 2022)

TikTok creator James Morrell (@jamesmorrell_) gained traction through comedy skits and documenting his life as a young man working as a barista and aspiring actor. When he started experiencing alopecia (later diagnosed with Crohn's disease) he documented his experience. Interviews and focus groups enable us to understand how men feel about their appearance in that one snapshot in time, which can give a binary impression that men are either concerned about their appearance or not. However, James' honest and open approach provided a valuable insight into the constant rollercoaster of emotions, with complex feelings fluctuating between positivity and despair. James continued to make comedy content in relation to his hair loss and raised a significant amount of money for Crohn's and Colitis UK through shaving his head live. However, his raw response to a comment accusing him of 'milking' his alopecia for content demonstrates the emotional impact hair loss can have on men as it challenges sense of identity and feelings of control:

> *Hey, I'm going through a lot recently. I've got quite a hefty weight pulling me down. And no, it's not my long brown luscious Scottish hair that I just spent a year growing weighing me down. No, it's actually quite the opposite. It's not having fucking consent before the powers that be [points up] deciding they were going to take this [hair] and run! Nobody asked me 'd'you wanna lose your hair?' cos that's a stupid fucking question, of course I didn't, of course I don't. I don't have a fucking choice so I'm slightly stressed, and I need an outlet. Cos if I don't let this shit out [spins camera to show river outside the house] I'll be swimming in the river. (@jamesmorrell_)*

In addition to loss of head hair, one study directly comparing men and women's experiences of chemotherapy-induced hair loss found a notable difference in men discussing hair loss from their bodies, whereas women did not address this. Modern beauty standards encourage women to remove hair from much of their body to appeal to a male gaze. However, the hairless body aesthetic is rarely a body standard that men aspire to, with a lack of hair associated with a pre-pubescent look. Men talked negatively about their hairless bodies using self-deprecating imagery such as "*a plucked chicken*" (Hilton et al., 2008) to describe themselves. One man who began a new relationship whilst experiencing chemotherapy-induced hair loss across his body described a feeling of discomfort. Although he explains that it's *not a deformity*, this is interestingly the word that comes to mind and provides an insight into how disconnected he feels from his body due to this loss of hair:

> *I mean there was literally just no hair on my body, full stop and it, it, it, it kind of felt very strange to be entering in a relationship and you know and entering a sexual relationship as well, with such a, a different body to the norm basically. I wouldn't say deformed because it wasn't, it's not, it's not a deformity ... it's just something different. (YPC20, chemotherapy-induced alopecia, UK)* (Hilton et al., 2008)

Facial hair is seemingly such a prominent marker of masculinity that it has been harnessed by men's charity Movember as part of their marketing campaign for men to grow a moustache throughout November to raise sponsorship money. Thus, although loss of facial hair wasn't discussed by all men (Trusson & Quincey, 2021) for those who did, there was a marked feeling of loss of masculinity throughout their narratives. Whilst some men missed the beard or moustache itself, Tristan expresses feeling infantilised by this loss of being able to shave his facial hair off:

> *I miss shaving ... it's like a manhood thing isn't it, shaving? Children don't shave. (Tristan, 41yrs, alopecia areata, UK)* (Zucchelli et al., 2022)

4.3 Clothing Choices

Due to physical changes to their bodies men often discussed having to make different clothing choices. This could be to accommodate things they were no longer able to do such as tying shoelaces or doing up buttons (due to limited dexterity), or to hide visible aspects of their condition. Whilst there is limited literature on the impact of disability on clothing choices, both men and women with rheumatoid arthritis have talked about the difficulty of finding footwear that is aesthetically acceptable to them, and the resulting consequences on clothing choices (Wilson et al., 2017). The men in both my rheumatoid arthritis and systemic sclerosis focus groups often discussed clothing choices in functional and practical rather than aesthetic terms. This could be due to the all-male focus group setting deterring talk of aesthetics, or the men in my studies may have simply been more concerned with function over style. The men also shared tips with each other for clothing and footwear options, which aligns with the idea that men build rapport and support each other through shared problem solving:

Chris *Although I did tie my own shoelaces today [laughs].*
Henry *I was about to say, you're the only person wearing shoes with laces. I can't wear them.*
Chris *But I swa-, I swapped those this morning for another pair, with a Velcro strap on them, so yes.*
George *I thank goodness for long handled shoehorns and brogues and slip on shoes. I've even managed to find some outdoor boots that you can slip on.*
(Focus group with men with systemic sclerosis, UK)

It's also important to highlight that beyond aesthetics and function, clothing can have cultural significance and personal importance. Samson describes feeling unable to wear his traditional clothing due to feeling too exposed. Thus, this impact of prostate cancer on his body image is also beginning to encroach on his ability to embrace his cultural identity:

> *I can't put on my beautiful Kente ntoma (traditional Ghanaian wear) because the catheter and urine bag will be seen by others. Also, wearing the Kente will expose my extreme weight loss. I need to wear something that can conceal it (catheter) and cover my entire body and not expose it too much. So, wearing my favourite Kente is out of the option. (Samson, prostate cancer, Ghanaian)* (Salifu et al., 2023)

4.4 The Loss of a Masculine Body

Men may desire a body that aligns with hegemonic masculine ideals of strength, power, and competence. This can mean having a large frame and/or a muscular physique with upper arm strength often being valued. Male bodies are important in constructing masculinity in male fitness spaces (Wagner, 2016). There is also a growing awareness that body dysmorphia and eating disorders are more common in men than previously acknowledged (Hendricks et al., 2023), demonstrating the value some men place on body image. Thus, despite (as mentioned earlier) men with systemic sclerosis reporting being generally unconcerned about visible facial differences, changes to their bodies were a different matter.

Men experienced weight and muscle loss due to systemic sclerosis. Some men initially described being satisfied with a small amount of weight loss. However, as this progressed, they were left with a body they no longer recognised. Chris (below) describes himself as under his *fighting weight*, which he uses as a turn of phrase rather than literally, yet this way of describing his smaller body hints at feeling a loss of physical power. It may also be a way of reframing body image issues in masculine terms, which may make it easier to discuss. Similarly, Jim and John describe themselves as '*weaker*'. Many of the men had noticeably monitored the changes to their bodies and were often able to list the difference in their weight since diagnosis:

> *No, I'm, I'm half to three quarters of a stone lighter than my fighting weight if you like so, no, that would be muscle loss, definitely. Yeah, I look in the mirror and think who's that? (Chris, 55yrs, systemic sclerosis, White British)*

Jim *Well I, I actually I thought, thought losing the 501bs as I was heavy I thought losing the 501bs would be a big benefit to me in walking and climbing stairs and doing these other things but it's not, I mean I'm, I'm weaker than I was ....*

John *Yeah, definitely weaker.*

Jim *... than I, er, I can't do as much as I did when I weighed 50llbs more.*

John *Yeah, the same way I, I started at about 235 and lost 50, so and again was in far, far better shape and condition than a, and stamina at 235 than I am down around 190 now, gaining some of it back, but ... Yeah, definitely haven't gained back any stamina or strength.*

(Focus group of men with systemic sclerosis, USA)

In contrast, Steve (below) discusses his difficulties with an increased appetite due to steroid tablets and talks about the importance to him of not gaining weight. Some men discussed a sense of achievement in reaching weight loss goals, until this became too rapid. Thus, a desirable male body may need a careful and individual balance of mass for a body that is big and strong, whilst not being overweight. Beyond body size and aspiring to a hegemonic body ideal, men's discomfort with a changing body size may relate to a desire for control over their own bodies:

> *I don't like being overweight, I just like … I have to seriously rein myself in otherwise I just eat everything that moves. (Steve, 44yrs, rheumatoid arthritis, White British)*

Whilst some men were keen to distance themselves from body image concerns, others explicitly recognised this as important to them. Derek (below) positions his weight concerns in relation to health and dismisses appearance concerns as feminine. This framing of weight as a health issue aligns with dominant masculine traits of taking responsibility. Thus, he can reject caring about body image as feminised, whilst still looking after his body. However, for other men sculpting their body image could itself be aligned to taking responsibility. Vegar (below) describes *building my body* implying an active role in reclaiming control over the way he looks. There may also be a cultural element to Vegar openly discussing his self-image, as hegemonic masculinity in Norway places emphasis on outdoor life and sports-related activities, which relates to the value he places on 'building' his body and keeping fit. The social and legal emphasis on gender egalitarianism in Norwegian culture may also contribute to hegemonic masculinity in Norway not being defined in opposition to values associated with femininity:

> *I think women are more conscious of their body weight than men … Cos of their appeal to men I think … How they look, men aren't as worried about how they look. … I think its health more than anything that would make [men] lose weight. (Derek, 76yrs, obese with knee osteoarthritis, White British)* (Toye et al., 2017)

> *I'm very satisfied. I put a lot of work into building my body … Not just for … not just for health, but also to build my self-image … Create more sense of achievement. And then everything good in life comes from that. (Vegar, bariatric surgery, Norwegian)* (Groven et al., 2015)

For many men a body diminished in size seemed to be experienced as a loss and they grieved for the body they used to know. A smaller framed body with muscle loss was often discussed by men in derogatory terms, making unfavourable comparisons to themselves. One man with systemic sclerosis described himself as "*just a bag of bones*" (James), whilst Opoku compares his body to that of a child suffering extreme malnourishment:

> *Indeed, I use to be a well-built handsome man. I've wasted and changed so much … look [showing his hair] it's sparse, and I look like a child with kwashiorkor [a malnourished child]. (Opoku, prostate cancer, Ghanaian)* (Salifu et al., 2023)

For many men it wasn't simply the difference in physical size that concerned them, loss of muscle mass and definition was a key factor. Beyond the appearance of muscle loss men were aware of the resulting loss of strength and abilities, which can have a marked impact on masculine identity (see Chap. 2):

Henry	*Yes, muscle weight I certainly have.*
George	*Mm. I lost a lot of weight, I think I lost five kilos and it's come, it came back a little bit I think I'm now, I lost four kilos or so, but my upper body strength is non-existent and, erm, I find it very difficult to get, get up off the floor.*
Henry	*Yeah, that's difficult.*
George	*Just not got the strength, it went overnight. It was amazing. (Focus group with men with systemic sclerosis, UK)*

Some men with long-term conditions experience bodily changes as not only a loss of masculine prowess but extending beyond this into a feminisation of their bodies. In addition to weight changes and decreased muscle mass, men undergoing treatment for prostate cancer can experience hot flushes and breast growth, which are associated with women's bodily experiences. Men expressed this not just as an unwelcome departure from masculine traits, but directly acknowledged this feminisation:

> *Hmm, I'm becoming a woman. After starting the chemo for some time, my breast had begun increasing just like that of ladies. If this should continue, it means I might need to wear a brassiere [he laughs]. (Nii, prostate cancer, Ghanaian)* (Salifu et al., 2023)

Bodily hair loss (previously discussed) was also related to body feminisation, which Lucian argues is potentially more important to gay men due to lazy stereotypes of gay men being effeminate. This also ties in with findings that gay men tend to aspire to a more muscular ideal than heterosexual men with self-esteem tied to body image satisfaction (Yelland & Tiggemann, 2003). Thus, it could be argued that retaining control over the masculinisation of their bodies could be more important to gay men in relation to building masculine capital (De Visser & McDonnell, 2013):

> *Being gay and people sometimes have the assumption that you're going to be effeminate, and then suddenly you've no hairs either as well then, in my mind, it makes a difference. (Lucian, 38yrs, alopecia areata, UK)* (Zucchelli et al., 2022)

Unsurprisingly, there was a marked impact on men who experienced changes to their genitalia, with many men describing this as emasculating. Men used self-deprecating language to describe their changed bodies ("*really shrivelled-up looking little penis*") (Oliffe, 2006) and express this feeling of body feminisation:

> *Well I must admit, that it took a lot of accepting. It took a lot of accepting to think that I was going to lose my manhood.' then it starts to dawn on you then: you are no longer you're half a man. (P8, penile cancer, UK)* (Bullen et al., 2010)

4.5 Living with a 'Women's Condition'

Both rheumatoid arthritis and systemic sclerosis are conditions that affect more women than men. Most of the men who took part in my focus groups were aware of this gender difference but didn't seem to consider this as having any impact on their sense of masculinity. In the below exchange Steve jokes about this, indicating they have a *feminine side*, but this is the closest any of the interactions came to acknowledging any feelings of feminisation due to the epidemiological gender split of their conditions:

Steve *And the amount of women that have it, unlike us, I didn't realise that it was something that wasn't just really common in men, it seems to be women get it as well.*

Henry *That surprised me that.*
CF *How does that feel that more women get it? Does that matter?*
Henry *I feel I can blame someone now!*
Steve *Maybe we're lucky, maybe we've got the feminine side, that's what it is.*
(Focus group with men with rheumatoid arthritis, UK)

However, the narrative in the breast cancer literature tells a different story. The whole marketing campaign around fundraising for breast cancer centres around the colour pink, generally associated with girls. The 'walk the walk' campaign encourages everyone taking part to wear decorated bras. In our common vocabulary we refer to women as having breasts and men as having chests. So, far beyond more women being diagnosed with breast cancer than men, the entire concept of having breast cancer is feminised through social constructs, and men were highly aware of this. Some highlighted the invisibility of their experience with male breast cancer being reasonably rare and seldom acknowledged in the media. For many, their masculine identity was affected through a breast cancer diagnosis, and worried that it challenged their masculine status:

Of all the cancers to get I had to get a bloody women's cancer. (Graham, breast cancer, UK). (Quincey et al., 2021)

I thought people would consider me less of a man because I had breast cancer. (P-21, breast cancer, USA) (Potter et al., 2023)

4.6 Other People's Perceptions

The men in my studies and throughout the long-term conditions literature discussed an awareness of how other people perceived them due to visible differences or disabilities, which impacted their self-image. Men were reluctant to accept an identity of being an invalid, and worried that other people would perceive them in this way. This isn't limited to men; previous interviews I conducted found women with rheumatoid arthritis were also concerned about other people's perceptions of them (Flurey et al., 2014b). However, there did seem to be a qualitative difference to these concerns with women being more focused on wanting people to understand their experiences, whereas men tended to not want to be recognised as disabled. When it comes to expressing pain, research has found for both men and women the presence of another person results in increasing pain tolerance. These differences are particularly high for men in the presence of male friends (Edwards et al., 2017). This indicates that both men and women experience a reluctance to demonstrate vulnerability in front of others, but it may be particularly important for men to perform masculinity in front of other men:

> *It's hard for people to understand, especially if you are quite young, why you can't do things, why you can't walk so fast and all that sort of stuff. (Charlotte, 37yrs, rheumatoid arthritis, White British)*

> *That's what I don't like is obviously being quite young and having it, they sort of… I don't know because sometimes I've had to use a walking stick and stuff like that, people look at me in the street and they're just horrified. It's just like why are you walking with a stick? (Steve 44yrs, rheumatoid arthritis, White British)*

Men also became aware of physical differences in their appearance when this caused concern about their health in other people. Some men resented the reminder of their condition due to other people's recoil at their changing body. Men with systemic sclerosis described colour changes in their fingers in the cold due to lack of blood flow and worried about causing unnecessary concern in people around them: "*[T]hey go the colour of a dead body, and everyone's looking at me saying what's wrong*" (Pete, 59yrs, systemic sclerosis, White British).

It could be argued that men are projecting their own awareness of visible differences onto the people around them. However, many men had experienced people commenting on their appearance, whether through genuine concern or male 'banter'. Perhaps due to societal expectations that men are not meant to be concerned with their appearance, men's bodies seem to be fair game for directly negative comments sometimes disguised as concern. However, this can contribute to a negative body image, and may reinforce the feeling of "*standing out from the herd*" (O'Brien et al., 2007):

Bill	*Yeah, 'why's your face so thin?', yeah, that's the one I would always get.*
CF	*Really, people actually comment?*
Bill	*Oh yeah, 'your face is thin', you know, 'we see the sockets in your cheeks where we didn't see them before'.*

John *Yeah that's what people at work noticed first, it was in the face, they said yeah ...*

Scott *Like I would get questions at work, people I didn't know, they were like, 'are you sick?' And it's kind of like, yeah, well actually I am [laughs], you know.*

(Focus group with men with systemic sclerosis, USA)

> *Actually, everyone at my work commented on it ... me being fat. I was ... my colleagues called me "the fat guy". ... And in a male-dominated workplace, it is kind of a rough style, and in such a climate being called the fat guy is normal. ... Instead of saying hello, they called you the fat guy ... it is kind of a jargon. ... And it was like that all the time. (Eirik, bariatric surgery, Norwegian)* (Groven et al., 2015)

Some men even discussed being judged on their appearance to the point where it affected their ability to work. In some cases, this may be due to a misplaced attempt by an employer to protect their employee from returning to work before they are well enough. However, it's important to remember (as discussed in Chap. 3) that maintaining paid work can have a marked positive impact on men's mental health and wellbeing. Whilst in the UK we are protected by the Equality Act (Equality Act, 2010) (with equivalent policy in many other countries), in some countries people are still directly or indirectly discriminated against due to visible differences and disability. Being judged as unfit for work based on appearance rather than ability is only likely to further impact mental wellbeing through challenging masculine self-image:

> *I find it a nightmare at the moment, only because of my weight loss through it. I didn't expect that, 'cause I was nearly like 12 ½ stone, now I'm struggling to keep seven stone. Which is a nightmare at the moment because, erm, work won't accept me back because like, they think I'm fragile, and frail because of the way I am in the office. (Alfie, systemic sclerosis, White British)*

> *When I was looking for a new job, I encountered great difficulties, for instance, while I was interviewed face to face. ... It was not easy to pass an interview; being treated with discrimination, being rejected, and sarcasm and spite were inevitable. In fact, people still hold a discriminatory attitude towards the population with facial disfigurement in our society. (oral cancer, Thai) (Hu et al.,* 2009*)*

In addition to not wanting to be negatively judged men were also aware of visible differences for the way they invited well-meaning but unwelcome pity or fuss. Visible differences served as a reminder to loved ones that men were living with a long-term condition. Men often described being infantilised by their mothers or partners but wanted to be seen and treated as normal. Support preferences will be discussed further in Chap. 9:

> *My mum drives down and says, 'okay what can we do' and I'm like, 'mum, you're stressing me out', and I don't want people to keep coming up to me every second, 'are you okay, are you okay'. Oh it drives me mad, it makes me even more angry, because I want to be seen normal, you know, come on talk about football or something, it's like 'how's your legs, how's your arms, how's your muscles. Oh man I really feel bad for you, I feel bad for you, let's try and do something', it's like, oh just please, leave me alone for a minute, let's have a normal talk. (Emil, 37, systemic sclerosis, Black British)*

Some men described concealing their condition to avoid unwelcome pity from strangers, or even to try and keep up appearances with those close to them. This is consistent with the idea that men may try to behave according to traditional masculine ideals and can subscribe to a learnt 'boy code' of hiding feelings of vulnerability (Pollack, 1998):

Jorge *I don't want the other people to feel like pity, right?*
Ted *Mm.*
Jorge *It's like, you know, I'm still normal right?*
Travis *Yeah.*
Jorge *So maybe that's why I don't, you know, I try to keep doing the same things, don't, don't demonstrate a limitation, just, you know, keep doing it and if I have to open this, okay I try to do it myself, you know, without showing that I'm struggling a little bit, er, but maybe from that point of view more, I, I don't want people to say, 'oh what's going on, tell me', it's like why, am I going to start telling you the whole story, like for what.*
(Focus group with men with systemic sclerosis, USA)

Finally, whilst much of this chapter has focused on visible differences it is worth highlighting that masculine self-image can also be challenged when their condition is invisible to others. In Western cultures, pain and disability are often constructed as something visible with pain expected to be accompanied by an obvious physical affliction or injury (Eccleston et al., 1997). Thus, invisible illnesses and their impact remain generally poorly understood. With the rise of social media, it is not uncommon to see people with hidden disabilities sharing videos of being challenged for using disabled toilets or parking spaces because they don't 'fit' the social expectation of what it looks like to be disabled (e.g., @karen_kevins on TikTok). Men discussed the awkwardness of not being able to give up their seats on public transport and feeling judged for not fulfilling the expectation of men to be chivalrous to women or the elderly. Thus, for some men once they started to develop visible signs of their condition, they found this easier to deal with than being unable to enact masculine roles and activities without a visible sign for people to understand:

> *And that's hard, like what he just said earlier, it's hard. I mean now I'm starting to show the physical signs of scleroderma, I'm starting to have the facial recognition but before, before I had my transplant and I couldn't breathe, and I had no lung, very very little lung capacity left, you couldn't tell I was sick. You know, 'he's not sick, you look …' Everybody at church and in the stores, 'oh you look so good, you look so good, you look so healthy', you know from the outside you look fine, but it's what you're going through that people don't understand that. You look fine. In their eyes you're fine. (Wade, 61yrs, systemic sclerosis, White American)*

4.7 Summary

Whilst societal assumptions still prevail that appearance and body image are issues that affect women more than men, men are also impacted by visible differences due to their condition. Some men withdraw from social activities such as avoiding fitness spaces to avoid exposing parts of their body. Men seemed to experience a particular impact on their masculine body image when their body reduced in size, and they lost muscle mass or perceived their bodies as becoming feminised. Retaining control over the masculinisation of their bodies may be particularly important to gay men, who may reject stereotypes of gay men as effeminate. Many men also tried to conceal their condition or visible differences resulting from their condition as they worried how others would perceive them. These worries were not unfounded with some men experiencing negative comments from others about their appearance, and even experiencing discrimination such as being judged unfit for work due to their appearance. Thus, clinicians should be aware that whilst men may play down body image concerns this can still have a marked impact on their quality of life, self-esteem, and wellbeing.

References

Bullen, K., Edwards, S., Marke, V., & Matthews, S. (2010). Looking past the obvious: Experiences of altered masculinity in penile cancer. *Psycho-Oncology, 19*(9), 933–940. https://doi.org/10.1002/pon.1642

De Visser, R. O., & McDonnell, E. J. (2013). "Man points": Masculine capital and young men's health. *Health Psychology, 32*(1), 5–14. https://doi.org/10.1037/A0029045

Eccleston, C., Williams, A. C., & Stainton Rogers, W. (1997). Patients' and professionals' understandings of the causes of chronic pain: Blame, responsibility and identity protection. *Social Science & Medicine, 45*(5), 699–709.

Edwards, R., Eccleston, C., & Keogh, E. (2017). Observer influences on pain: An experimental series examining same-sex and opposite-sex friends, strangers, and romantic partners. *Pain, 158*(5), 846–855. https://doi.org/10.1097/J.PAIN.0000000000000840

Equality Act, c. 15 (2010). https://www.legislation.gov.uk/ukpga/2010/15/contents

Flurey, C., Morris, M., Richards, P., Hughes, R., & Hewlett, S. (2014b). "It's like a juggling act": Rheumatoid Arthritis patient perspectives on daily life and flare whilst on current treatment regimes. *Rheumatology, 53*(4), 696–703.

Gentili, C., McClean, S., Hackshaw-McGeagh, L., Bahl, A., Persad, R., & Harcourt, D. (2019). Body image issues and attitudes towards exercise amongst men undergoing androgen deprivation therapy (ADT) following diagnosis of prostate cancer. *Psycho-Oncology, 28*(8), 1647–1653. https://doi.org/10.1002/pon.5134

Groven, K., Galdas, P., & Solbrække, K. (2015). Becoming a normal guy: Men making sense of long-term bodily changes following bariatric surgery. *International Journal of Qualitative Studies on Health and Well-Being, 10*(1). https://doi.org/10.3402/qhw.v10.29923

Hendricks, E., Jenkinson, E., Falconer, L., & Griffiths, C. (2023). How effective are psychosocial interventions at improving body image and reducing disordered eating in adult men? A systematic review. *Body Image, 47*(101612). https://doi.org/10.1016/j.bodyim.2023.08.004

Hilton, S., Hunt, K., Emslie, C., Salinas, M., & Ziebland, S. (2008). Have men been overlooked? A comparison of young men and women's experiences of chemotherapy-induced alopecia. *Psych-Oncology, 17*(6), 577–583. https://doi.org/10.1002/pon.1272

Hu, T. W., Cooke, M., & McCarthy, A. (2009). A qualitative study of the experience of oral cancer among Taiwanese men. *International Journal of Nursing Practice, 15*(4), 326–333. https://doi.org/10.1111/J.1440-172X.2009.01759.X

Mental Health Foundation. (2023). *Millions of men in the UK affected by body image issues—Mental Health Foundation survey*. https://www.mentalhealth.org.uk/about-us/news/millions-men-uk-affected-body-image-issues-mental-health-foundation-survey

O'Brien, R., Hart, G. J., &; Hunt, K. (2007). "Standing out from the herd": Men renegotiating masculinity in relation to their experience of illness. *International Journal of Men's Health, 6*(3), 178–200.

Oliffe, J. (2006). Embodied masculinity and androgen deprivation therapy. *Sociology of Health & Illness, 28*(4), 410–432. https://doi.org/10.1111/J.1467-9566.2006.00499.X

Pollack, W. S. (1998). *Real boys: Rescuing our sons from the myths of boyhood*. Henry Holt and Company.

Potter, A. M., Bentz, B., Crue, L., Leiby, S., Bashi, S., Maguire, K., Meyers, J., & Mieczkowski, K. (2023). Men's lived experiences of breast cancer and changes in occupation. *Occupational Therapy International*. https://doi.org/10.1155/2023/9641922

Quincey, K., Williamson, I., & Wildbur, D. (2021). Men with breast cancer and their encounters with masculinity: An interpretative phenomenological analysis using photography. *Psychology of Men and Masculinity, 22*(4), 690–703. https://doi.org/10.1037/MEN0000344

Rennie, C., Stoddart, K., & Hubbard, G. (2018). A new normal: Reconciling change in appearance and function for men with head and neck cancer. *Cancer Nursing Practice, 17*(5). https://doi.org/10.7748/cnp.2018.e1449

Salifu, Y., Almack, K., & Caswell, G. (2023). 'Out of the frying pan into the fire': A qualitative study of the impact on masculinity for men living with advanced prostate cancer. *Palliative Care and Social Practice, 17*. https://doi.org/10.1177/26323524231176829/

Toye, F., Room, J., & Barker, K. L. (2017). Do I really want to be going on a bloody diet? Gendered narratives in older men with painful knee osteoarthritis. *Disability and Rehabilitation, 40*(16), 1914–1920. https://doi.org/10.1080/09638288.2017.1323017

Trusson, D., & Quincey, K. (2021). Breast cancer and hair loss: Experiential similarities and differences in men's and women's narratives. *Cancer Nursing, 44*(1), 62–70.

Wagner, P. (2016). Picture perfect bodies: Visualizing hegemonic masculinities produced for/by male fitness spaces. *International Journal of Men's Health, 15*(3), 235–258.

Wilson, O., Kirwan, J., Dures, E., Quest, E., & Hewlett, S. (2017). The experience of foot problems and decisions to access foot care in patients with rheumatoid arthritis: A qualitative study. *Journal of Foot and Ankle Research, 10*(1), 1–11. https://doi.org/10.1186/S13047-017-0188-3

Yelland, C., & Tiggemann, M. (2003). Muscularity and the gay ideal: Body dissatisfaction and disordered eating in homosexual men. *Eating Behaviors, 4*(2), 107–116. https://doi.org/10.1016/S1471-0153(03)00014-X

Zucchelli, F., Sharratt, N., Montgomery, K., & Chambers, J. (2022). Men's experiences of alopecia areata: A qualitative study. *Health Psychology Open, 1–13.* https://doi.org/10.1177/20551029221121524

CHAPTER 5

Sex and Intimacy

"It's important that they ask the question first, 'cause it's a little embarrassing"

According to World Health Organisation (2023b) *"[A] central aspect of being human throughout life encompasses sex, gender identities and roles, sexual orientation, eroticism, pleasure, intimacy and reproduction"*. It should hardly be surprising that sex is an important component of wellbeing, yet when it comes to people with long-term conditions, sex and intimacy is often overlooked, ignored, or dismissed. The reasons for this are likely multifaceted. Sex is still widely considered a taboo topic in many cultures and social settings, which can cause us to feel embarrassed raising the subject, or to worry that we will cause embarrassment in the person we're talking to. This social taboo may be enhanced when thinking about sex in people with long-term conditions as the social construction promoted by the beauty industry is that sexual beings are physically able beings. In pornography, disabled bodies tend to be included as a 'kink' rather than as sexual beings in their own right. The lack of focus on sex and intimacy in people with long-term conditions may also be a product of the (conscious or unconscious) bias from an outsider perspective that with all the physical symptoms of a long-term condition (e.g., pain, fatigue) people would have more to worry about than their sex lives. However, my focus groups with men with systemic sclerosis and findings from the wider literature demonstrate that this is far from true.

C. Flurey, *Talking Men's Health*,
https://doi.org/10.1007/978-3-031-62593-0_5

5.1 The Importance of Sex

Systemic sclerosis is a condition that affects blood flow to the extremities, and men have one extremity that's arguably more important to them than all the others. Erectile dysfunction is therefore a potential symptom of systemic sclerosis and so I had planned to directly ask about this issue in my focus groups. However, it was rarely necessary as participants were often forthcoming in raising these issues themselves. Whilst not all men with long-term conditions are affected by sex and intimacy issues, of those men who are many highlighted this as a key issue. In my focus groups, the majority of men raised this as the thing that bothers them most about living with systemic sclerosis:

> *It's upsetting, it, it's upsetting, that's very much it, that's, if you said to me, 'what's the worst?', making love. (Karim, systemic sclerosis, British Asian)*

To put this into context of how important sex and intimacy is to these men's quality of life, it is important to remember that systemic sclerosis is a potentially life-limiting condition with an average life expectancy of five years from diagnosis. These men experienced an array of physical symptoms, some with internal organ involvement, and many worried about their mortality (see Chap. 6). Yet often when I asked, "If there was one thing you would change about your condition what would it be?", the response was related to sex and intimacy rather than mortality. In contrast, interviews with men with prostate cancer found that although they struggled to come to terms with impotency issues, they prioritised their mortality over their sex lives:

> *If you are alive you can do whatever you can do; if you are dead then you can't do anything. So the first objective is to be alive. (Patrick, prostate cancer, Anglo-Australian)* (Oliffe, 2005)

Men with prostate cancer are in a very different position of needing to make a cost-benefit analysis between sex and mortality through making a choice to have life-saving treatment that may cause erectile dysfunction. For these men with prostate cancer their mortality was an imminent threat that had to be addressed. However, for men with systemic sclerosis, sex and intimacy may regularly affect their quality of life or relationships and may pose an immediate threat to their masculinity. Further, ignoring or dismissing potential threats to mortality to focus on immediate concerns may be protective. For most men with prostate cancer, once the immediate threat to life was addressed, erectile dysfunction and loss of libido were discussed as the worst adverse effects of their treatment.

Whichever way we look at this, if mortality is the one thing prioritised over sex and intimacy then this is clearly a crucial aspect of men's experiences of living with a long-term condition.

5.2 Erectile Dysfunction and Beyond: Impact of Illness on Sexual Performance

Men experience issues such as inability to maintain erections sufficiently for penetration, and/or a diminished libido, difficulty ejaculating or decreased ejaculations, and less intense orgasms. Whilst erectile dysfunction is perhaps the most obvious symptom that springs to mind when we think about impact on sexual performance, there are many other ways that men talk about long-term conditions affecting their sex lives.

Beyond erectile dysfunction, men talk about sex being impacted by specific physical symptoms associated with their condition. In men with systemic sclerosis, this included pain, lack of energy, breathlessness, and tightened skin around their penis. Men with inflammatory arthritis report pain and swollen joints causing sex to become less spontaneous or less frequent (Perez-Garcia et al., 2021). Some physical symptoms can particularly impact on preferred roles in gay sex, as this man with diabetes explains:

> *As a diabetic, I sometimes suffer from a Candidiasis [thrush] in my buttocks. This makes it impossible to be the 'bottom' in anal intercourse. (Ben, 28yrs, diabetes, USA)* (Jowett et al., 2011)

Men with systemic sclerosis in my own focus groups and men with long-term conditions throughout the wider literature discuss the impact of illness on their libido. This can be due to specific physical symptoms such as pain, the overall feeling of being unwell, or from side effects of medication:

> *For me it, it's the libido was the change, I, I don't have an issue with erectile dysfunction, touch wood and sildenafil [also known by the brand name Viagra] obviously helps with that [laughs], erm, particularly I had, erm, a whole load*

of pulsed Cyclophosphamide [intravenous chemotherapy drug] and at that point my libido did tank massively compared to what it was. (James, 44yrs, systemic sclerosis, White British)

In addition to the impact of physical symptoms on their sex lives, men described an additional psychological impact. They explained that worries about their sexual performance could itself impact that performance. Men in both my own studies and the wider literature reported ongoing sex and intimacy issues affecting their confidence:

Karim *And, the, the problem is, is if it's happening for a month, two months or three months, then you lack confidence [laughs].*
Emil *Mentally, mentally ...*
Karim *You're worrying it's going to happen just when you, you're about to penetrate, or while you're in there [laughs] ...*
Emil *That's it.*
(Focus group with men with systemic sclerosis, UK)

5.3 Impact on Masculinity

With sexual prowess being intricately linked with masculinity, men often describe a marked psychological impact of issues with sex and intimacy on their masculine identity. As discussed throughout this book there are multiple ways in which long-term conditions impact masculinity, such as losing strength and bulk (Chap. 4) or being unable to fulfil traditionally masculine roles in the family (Chap. 2). So, on top of difficulties with sex affecting masculinity, many men report a vicious cycle with feelings of diminished masculinity from multiple disease-related causes also affecting their confidence with sex.

Throughout the literature across multiple conditions, countries, and sexualities men made connections between masculinity and having a functioning penis. Men with prostate cancer used terms such as *"mutilated"*, *"incomplete"*, *"unmaly, invisible, and worthless"* (Alexis & Worsley, 2018) to describe this loss of function. Penis functioning was viewed as an integral part of masculine identity with any impairment experienced as a loss of that identity:

> *Well, most people feel, it's a major loss of manhood. A man is no longer a man if he is not able to function. I think it's the way we were brought up. Most of us feel that we're no longer a man, if you're not able to do that. (62yrs, moderate erectile dysfunction, Chinese)* (Low et al., 2009)

In focus groups with gay men experiencing sexual difficulties, an interesting contrast was drawn. Erectile dysfunction was described as being "*seen as there is something wrong with me*", whilst experiencing pain during receptive anal sex "*isn't your fault … these things just happen*" (McDonagh et al., 2017). This highlights how a phallocentric model of sex is often dominant across constructions of masculinity, with a penis that functions as desired being intricately linked to hegemonic masculine ideals (Connell, 2005).

The following interaction between men with systemic sclerosis in the USA from one of my focus groups highlights the psychological impact of erectile dysfunction to these men's wellbeing and sense of self. They discuss the burden of being unable to 'perform', and amongst many other physical symptoms of systemic sclerosis they focus on erectile dysfunction as the issue assessed as a 'serious problem':

CF	*So coming back to, you said sex was a really important part of life that you're missing now, is that something that other people relate to, is that a big loss for everyone else?*
Wade	*Yes.*
Jacob	*Absolutely, yes.*
Wade	*Most definitely, when you can't perform, you can't perform and it, it takes a toll on you.*
Liam	*[…] that was one of the first indicators to me that something was wrong was I could no longer, er, get an erection and that occurred within the span of like, wow, it was like fire, it was like one to two months […] So I had a problem [laughs] and personally I felt I had a serious problem.*
Hank	*It is a serious problem.*
Liam	*And it affects you, as a guy.*
	(Focus group with men with systemic sclerosis, USA) (Flurey et al., 2022)

A common social construction in heterosexual relationships is that the man should be the one to take control, and perhaps be the more active partner in bed. As this quote from Emil demonstrates, those men whose long-term condition affected their ability to demonstrate this physical prowess experienced a negative impact on their self-esteem and found themselves questioning their self-worth:

> *[Sighs] oh it just feels like you're not there and that's why I had to get all these devices just to try and work, and get going [laughs] and my wife as well, 'cause I can't, I can't even get into a position 'cause I get cramp and I'm so stiff I can't move, so it's like, oh what good am I? You know, that's what it feels like, I can't even make love to you, I can't even get into a position, I can't move, I get cramp all down my legs and all down my back and all of it's gone, 'cause I'm in so much pain. I was like, okay, I can't do this. I just have to lay there trying to stretch it out and obviously the mood's gone and everything's gone, it's just frustration, it's so unbelievable. (Emil, 37yrs, systemic sclerosis, Black British)*

In gay relationships, some men defined themselves by their preferred sexual roles and positions (i.e., "top" referring to those who engage in the penetrative or 'insertive' role during sexual activity; "bottom" referring to those who engage in the receptive role; and "versatile" or "switch" referring to those who engage in both roles). For those gay men who were unable to adopt their preferred sexual role they explained that not only would their masculine identity be compromised but also their identity as a gay man:

> *[A] loss of identity because, like, they can't regard themselves as an active gay man. (Cormac, 30yrs, Irish)* (McDonagh et al., 2017)

5.4 Impact on Relationships

Men are often stereotyped as only thinking of their own pleasure when it comes to sex. However, the narratives from men with long-term conditions throughout the literature indicate that men's primary concern is often the impact on their relationships. Men discuss worrying about whether they are satisfying their wives, and whether their wives felt rejected or unattractive. The below extract describes these concerns and demonstrates how men were able to share these worries with each other:

Emil *Erm, and as I said for me the main thing is making love because I feel I'm upsetting her …*

All *Mm.*
Karim *... because she can't get the enjoyment she deserves in that area. That, that's the thing.*
(Focus group with men with systemic sclerosis, UK)

The following quote from interviews with men on how they perceive erectile dysfunction illustrates how concerns about being unable to sexually satisfy partners can challenge men's sense of value to their relationship. Of course men bring more to a marriage than their sexual prowess, and women value other qualities beyond sexual satisfaction. However, this participant's description of being unable to function properly as a husband demonstrates the value placed on performing sexually for reinforcing their self-esteem and self-worth:

> *I still feel very frustrated that I am unable to really function properly as a husband ... to give my wife full sexual satisfaction she would expect from a husband. (59yrs, mild erectile dysfunction, Chinese)* (Low et al., 2009)

Throughout the literature men with long-term conditions discuss experiencing strains on their relationship through losing the closeness that comes from intimacy. They are also aware of the impact on their wives of having to support them through the psychological impact of impotency issues. Men in long-term relationships or marriages often discussed feeling grateful for having this solid grounding to build on and over time were able to develop mutual coping strategies and understanding:

> *This is the emotional test of a relationship really because, er, then if the intimacy is a little bit lost then you, you kind of think, well I've lost that, no matter where you stand in the world, that, that's detrimental to your relationship because the intimacy's lost. (Paul, 52yrs, systemic sclerosis, White British)*

Hank *It definitely has a strain on any relationship, er, I would think. It did for me.*
Liam *Sure, I think, erm, the, the issues are internal for men, when it first starts out, again I'm talking for myself so there's a lot of problems mentally starting out that you have to overcome and have to deal with and that took several months for me to kind of figure out and work through but at the time I had been married for, oh let me see,*

> *maybe 18 years, 18, 19 years so I've got a spouse that was very understanding, you know, erm, and I had that going for me, but still again that doesn't matter at the time, as a guy. I've got, I've got a problem.*
> *(Focus group with men with systemic sclerosis, USA)*

Some men expressed concerns about their partners going elsewhere if they were unable to satisfy them. In my focus groups in the UK this issue was raised through humour as demonstrated by Frank (below). This could be interpreted as male 'banter' as part of group bonding in the male focus group setting. However, humour can also be used effectively to mask and protect from underlying worries that we may not even feel able to directly admit to ourselves. Other men felt able to discuss these concerns much more directly. The below excerpt from an interview with a man with diabetes in sub-Saharan Africa demonstrates the depth of these feelings. Whilst he starts with a focus on his wife looking elsewhere sexually, he continues on to demonstrate he's worried about the greater impact of losing his wife from his life:

> *They might think well I'm going somewhere else, you know, the milkman [laughs] (Frank, 64yrs, systemic sclerosis, White British)* (Flurey et al., 2022)

> *I worry she might look elsewhere to satisfy her needs. … I worry about it every day because I don't know how I'd cope without her. Really. She helps me with everything. Does everything to take care of me. (type 2 diabetes, sub-Saharan Africa)* (Cooper et al., 2018)

According to these interviews with men with diabetes in sub-Saharan Africa, concerns about infidelity are not necessarily a one-way street. Many of these men found it difficult to discuss sexual problems with their partners. This left their partners feeling suspicious that they were having their sexual needs satisfied outside of the relationship. Many of these men described being falsely accused of infidelity, which they expressed as hurtful and distressing:

> *It's causing problems for me and my wife. She thinks I'm having sex with other women. …- When my wife sees my performance she says things like: 'Why you so weak? Have been bewitched by another lady? Did you have sex during the day?*

You think I'm a fool?' (type 2 diabetes, sub-Saharan Africa) (Cooper et al., 2018)

In contrast to impotence causing partners to worry that men are getting sexual satisfaction elsewhere, this man expresses concerns that taking medication for erectile dysfunction may cause their partners to worry that this will lead to promiscuity:

> *The other thing is that women also believe that if you have a loaded gun [erect penis], you would want to shoot. If they are not around, they'll be worried you'll be shooting someone else. (62yrs, moderate erectile dysfunction, Chinese)* (Low et al., 2009)

Many men express a desire for their partners to better understand their experiences. Emil (below) suggests it would be helpful for support to be available for couples. This could help partners to better understand the issues men with long-term conditions are facing in relation to sex and intimacy issues, and to enable partners to discuss their own thoughts and feelings in relation to these issues:

> *I would love my wife to talk to someone about this … but she don't know who to talk to, so maybe if there was a class where you were to talk to us as a couple, then she could get to understand me 'cause she probably feel like I'm moaning at her, 'why haven't we made love in so long?', 'cause obviously she goes into defence mode and 'cause I'm struggling physically, I'm frustrated, right, you know, I come to her with my frustration and anger and obviously she just tucks in, but talking to a doctor about it, it might help her understand, 'cause she doesn't have anyone to talk to. (Emil, 37yrs, systemic sclerosis, Black British)*

It's important to note that too often approaches to understanding sex and intimacy come from a perspective of patients being married or in committed relationships. However, sex and intimacy issues also affect single people, whether they are seeking a life partner or pursuing more casual arrangements. Whenever I've read advice provided through clinics or patient charities on having sex with a long-term condition, I've often wondered how this would work in the context of a one night stand—and of course this isn't an experience that should be denied to those with long-term conditions. Sex and intimacy when single with a long-term condition presents quite different but nonetheless important challenges. Single men in both my own studies and the wider literature talk about giving up on pursuing new sexual partners. As this man with inflammatory arthritis (below) describes, explaining sex and intimacy issues to a potential new partner can be difficult. In this man's experience it led to the relationship ending before it had begun:

> *Erectile dysfunction is a big issue for me. I still like to chase women. I have a girlfriend, I don't have a wife. It's a girlfriend, she comes and goes. She does whatever she wants, I do whatever I want. I like chasing women but I no longer do that, 'cause there's no sense in it. (Hank, systemic sclerosis, 62yrs, White American)*

> *I met a girl last year … and I didn't damn well know how I was going to bring it up because I knew he wasn't working as well as he had before, "John Thomas" … but it petered out … because I explained to her that I had a bit of a problem with erections … he's not dead … it works, of course, but … dammit'. (47yrs, inflammatory arthritis, Sweden)* (Östlund et al., 2015)

This issue may be even more pronounced in the gay dating scene, as explained by Colin (below). He describes how in his experience there is more of an expectation for the first date to lead to sex than in the heterosexual dating scene. This adds additional pressure from the very start of an interaction, and he describes how this led to him feeling unable to talk to a man who he was highly attracted to due to fears of being unable to perform and the impact on his reputation in the local scene:

> *I couldn't even talk to him. I was too frightened because I wouldn't want somebody on our local scene to know that erm, I couldn't rise to the occasion. And that's the one problem with gay life … in heterosexuality, you meet on another occasion and you go out and you go for dinner or for whatever and you chat to them. It's a long time before you actually got into bed, but the gay life was never like that, that was almost always the first time you meet. So that was terrifying me I couldn't do it. (Colin, 62yrs, diabetes, USA)* (Jowett et al., 2011)

5.5 Whatever It Takes: Pills, Porn, and Pumps

Men talked about trying anything and everything they could think of to help with sex and intimacy issues. Men with systemic sclerosis were often already taking medication such as sildenafil to manage circulation issues of their condition, which is more commonly known by its brand name Viagra—a drug used to help manage erectile dysfunction. However, medication rarely comes alone without side effects, and Paul described how this had a negative impact on his mood, which led to changing medications to one that was less effective at controlling erectile dysfunction:

> *It's hard to get sexually, so readily sexually aroused, it's hard, there's no doubt about that. Erm, I, I was initially on sildenafil to help with blood circulation for my hands, obviously and also it has an effect on your sexual performance, as it were ... but I got very irritable and unusually angry ... and the missus noticed the difference in my moods, so I switched from sildenafil Viagra, to, er, losartan potassium, losartan ... Erm, and that's okay. It's improved my hand circulation a little bit for the, for the Reynaud's so they've changed the medication that took place fairly in, fairly shortly into my diagnosis, so that's there but, er, it is harder to get an erection, it's harder to, it's harder to ejaculate. You know, even if I masturbated, I couldn't ejaculate, I thought what on earth's going on here. (Paul, 52yrs, systemic sclerosis, White British)*

Due to these concerns about side effects, a study with Thai men with diabetes found traditional medicines such as red ginseng extract were sometimes preferred to Western medicine (Thongtang et al., 2021). In the UK we rarely have to concern ourselves with the cost of prescribed medication as we pay a flat prescription cost with some patients exempt from costs. However, in other countries (such as Malaysia, exemplified by the below quote) the cost of medication for erectile dysfunction was prohibitive for men being able to access this treatment, and some explained that they seek out cheaper alternatives:

> *38 ringgit [US$10]. As big as this ... like the shape of this nail. But ... Viagra had two factories, the one that I'm consuming is from Germany. Another one is made in India. The one made in India is cheaper. (51yrs, moderate erectile dysfunction, Malay)* (Low et al., 2009)

Men discussed using sex toys or sexual aids in an effort to improve their sexual performance. Men throughout the wider literature discussed the use of foreplay and oral sex to satisfy their partners, which enabled them to feel a sense of sexual accomplishment in helping their partner achieve orgasm:

> *I do foreplay and sometimes I do oral sex to please my partner sexually. Because I figure if I can make her orgasm first then she is satisfied. (diabetes, Northern Thai)* (Thongtang et al., 2021)

This wasn't discussed in my own studies, which could be due to the focus group setting inhibiting the sharing of more intimate details, or due to feeling less comfortable with myself a female facilitator. However, this didn't prohibit men from discussing the use of sex toys and aids. To help them stimulate or maintain an erection some men discussed using pornographic media, and some had tried penis pumps. These had varied results with men sometimes expressing embarrassment at the need for these aids, and others felt frustration at the lack of effectiveness:

> *I've got a pump, I've got all these, I even bought toys and everything, I tried to work round the situation just to try and make something work, and it's crazy, the procedure you have to do to try and get a normal erection. (Emil, 37yrs, systemic sclerosis, Black British)*

> *Well, you have a highly inflated penis. Unfortunately it's all volume, no rigidity. It is normal erect size, but frightfully red looking and it is quite painful, but all of that would be okay if you had a degree of rigidity, so the truth is it has not allowed us to have penetrative sex. It is not rigid enough to do that. (Ben, prostate cancer, Anglo-Australian)* (Oliffe, 2005)

5.6 Don't Ask, Don't Tell: Healthcare Professionals Need to Ask About Sex

Systemic sclerosis is a condition that affects blood flow to the extremities, making erectile dysfunction a common symptom. So, I was surprised to find that for the men in my focus groups this had rarely been addressed by clinicians unless the men raised the issue themselves. None of the men remembered this being discussed with them at diagnosis. These men with systemic sclerosis explained they had to work out for themselves that erectile dysfunction was a part of their condition:

Wade *Well I had figured it out, I had not talked about it to my physician but I had read and I, I joined, erm, a scleroderma foundation and I used to get the, well I do get the newsletter and I, I was reading articles where the arteries are hardened and by the arteries hardening the walls of the artery get thicker, thus restricting the blood flow, so I figured well, I mean, it's all about blood flow so I kind of put two and two together, you know,*

CF *You had to figure it out on your own?*

Wade *I had to figure it out through my own self-study.*
CF *Mm, is that other people's experience or … Is this something that is discussed with your clinicians?*
Liam *I don't remember it ever being brought, up, not that I recall.*
Hank *It wasn't brought up for myself.*
Liam *And I wasn't saying much about it at the time [laughs] either, to be honest. You know I was not ready to open up about it, so.*
(Focus group of men with systemic sclerosis, USA) (Flurey et al., 2022)

This lack of discussion from clinicians seems particularly marked in a condition that affects blood flow to the extremities. However, this lack of focus on sex and intimacy in consultations is a recurring theme across the long-term conditions literature for both men and women across multiple long-term conditions, and in multiple countries. Men with inflammatory arthritis report difficulties accessing information related to sex. They often found online information inadequate and healthcare professionals too busy to address the issue (Perez-Garcia et al., 2021). A study conducted in Denmark found 93.5% of women and 85.5% of men with rheumatoid arthritis had not discussed sexual issues with healthcare professionals in the preceding five years (Bay et al., 2020). Additionally, in cultures that highly value reproduction, sex and intimacy issues may be discussed in younger men but are ignored in those men over traditional child-bearing age (Hayashi et al., 2023).

The strong language used by the following participants in relation to this highlights the frustration at such a key element of quality of life and wellbeing going unaddressed:

> *Not even a hint of a question on your sex life, on erections or anything. I think that's crap! (47yrs, inflammatory arthritis, Sweden)* (Östlund et al., 2015)

> *If you can talk so much about smoking and wrong food and unsaturated fatty acids, why the hell should we not be able to talk about these things? (66yrs, erectile dysfunction in cardiac rehabilitation, Denmark)* (Gerbild et al., 2021)

As men often value seeking information to become experts in their condition, an argument could be made that there is something empowering in them doing their own research. However, it is important to remember that not everyone has the same literacy or health literacy levels. Hank explains that he is illiterate; he therefore didn't have access to the same research tools as his contemporaries in the focus group. Imagine for a moment having been diagnosed with a life-changing condition, and a few months later you start to experience erectile dysfunction. Your clinicians discussed all sorts of other physical symptoms with you but didn't mention this, and you're not able to quickly check in with Dr Google. You don't know if this is a symptom of your new condition or yet another issue to cope with on top. It's so important that healthcare professionals don't shy away from discussing sex and intimacy issues with patients:

> *I was surprised that the scleroderma affected that. I was really surprised that it affected that, you know, but I'm illiterate, most of y'all probably can read. I don't do with computers, most of y'all probably can go on the internet and find out all kind of interesting cures that's been come up with. (Hank, 62yrs, systemic sclerosis, White American)* (Flurey et al., 2022)

Further, cultural beliefs can play a key role in contributing to health beliefs and understanding. These examples from men in Malaysia and India with erectile dysfunction demonstrate the importance of healthcare professionals discussing sex and intimacy issues to help men understand the cause and ensure they can seek appropriate medical support:

> *This is done by the 'bomoh' [Malay traditional health practitioner], he can shut our sexual desire, kill our desire. (55yrs, moderate erectile dysfunction, Malay)* (Low et al., 2009)

> *You see, it all depends how much he makes use of this [penis]. The more you use, the faster it [penis] deteriorates. (67yrs, severe erectile dysfunction, Indian)* (Low et al., 2009)

A systematic review of qualitative studies with healthcare professionals in the UK found barriers to discussing sex and intimacy issues included worries about "opening up a can of worms" if they asked about issues that they lacked the time or skills to address in clinic. Healthcare professionals expressed concerns that it wouldn't be fair to a patient to bring up sex and intimacy issues if they were unable to deal with them. Social taboos around sex were also an issue with their own personal discomfort in raising the topic as well as worries about causing offence to patients by being intrusive or inappropriate. Healthcare professionals also felt they lacked knowledge and training (Dyer & das Nair, 2013). This aligns with research with multidisciplinary healthcare professionals in rheumatic diseases who report they seldom discuss sexual health with patients, despite considering it important. However, they were more likely to feel comfortable enough to discuss these issues if they had received relevant training in sexual health than staff without such training (Helland et al., 2013).

Healthcare professionals felt particularly ill-equipped to discuss sex and intimacy issues in relation to intellectual disabilities, LGBTQIA+ issues, and older people, which they reported were only briefly covered in their curriculum, if not absent altogether. Most were keen to increase their knowledge about other communities' sexual practice and lifestyles. Some GPs reported feeling less comfortable discussing sex and intimacy issues with opposite-gender patients, which was partly due to concerns this could "sexualize the consultation". However, gender was not cited as a barrier by the majority of healthcare professionals (Dyer & das Nair, 2013). Providing training to empower healthcare professionals to discuss sexual health issues with patients that takes into account a variety of demographics, lifestyles, and cultures should therefore be a key consideration across long-term conditions.

Some healthcare professionals expressed the view that sex and intimacy issues are not directly a medical issue and are beyond their professional role. This attitude was also experienced by men throughout the long-term conditions literature, with one participant's urologist telling him during a pre-surgery meeting for prostate cancer treatment:

> *This is not my job to make sure you are going to have sexual functioning. My job is to save your life. (Tony, 55yrs, prostate cancer, Canada)* (Letts et al., 2010)

Despite clinicians often not being forthcoming about discussing sex, the men with systemic sclerosis in my focus groups who had been diagnosed for some time did feel able to bring these issues up to their clinical teams. However, they also note that they would prefer their clinical teams to ask about it themselves as they find it embarrassing:

CF *So, would you prefer if your clinician raised it for you, for you to be able to talk about it?*
Liam *Sure.*

Wade *If they would have arose with the question then there would have been a response, do you see what I'm saying. So yeah, I think it's important that they ask the question first, 'cause it's a little embarrassing.*

Hank *It is kind of embarrassing, it's an embarrassing thing for a man, maybe not a woman, I don't know.*

(Focus group with men with systemic sclerosis, USA)

It's important to remember that due to their long-standing relationship with their clinical team, these patients may be more comfortable than the general population would be about discussing issues such as erectile dysfunction with their clinicians. Frank's quote highlights this, explaining that whilst he might be comfortable to discuss sex now, he certainly wouldn't have been when he was younger:

> *20 years ago I might have been reluctant to bring it up, I might have been embarrassed I just don't know. Er, and it's embarrassing talking about it with blokes, never mind a lady [CF—researcher] in here, but, er, I don't know, I think it would have been good for somebody to mention it right at the beginning. Now I don't know if it affects everybody with systemic sclerosis ... but I think it would be good just to highlight it, that it's a great possibility. (Frank, 64yrs, systemic sclerosis, White British)* (Flurey et al., 2022)

Interestingly, one of the focus group participants expressed how he was worried about whether erectile dysfunction would be discussed or not during the focus group. This was clearly an important issue to him that he wanted to discuss, but he worried about being the one to have to raise this, particularly within a group of other men. This highlights the importance of clinicians raising these issues because even when men are prepared to bring them up themselves it may cause them unnecessary stress and worry:

Wade *I was wondering if that topic [erectile dysfunction] was going to be brought up today and how are we going to address it if it was and I, I thought about that, you know, would that topic be, since we're all men, would that topic be brought up, or, or am I the only one with that situation. So that crossed my mind.*

CF *Was it a worry, was it worrying that it might come up?*

Wade *Yes, yes.*

CF *Because ...?*

Wade *'Cause it's like do I bring it up, if no one brings it up do I bring it up? It was something I'd thought about.*
(Focus group with men with systemic sclerosis, USA)

5.7 Talking to Men About Sex and Intimacy

Even within just my own focus groups there was a wide range of ways men discussed sex and intimacy with some prepared to be quite direct with the conversation. However, others indirectly sought permission to discuss sex, waiting until they were confident I understood their implication before opening up:

CF *So what would you say is the worst part of, erm, systemic sclerosis, what's the one symptom or impact on your life you'd get rid of if you could?*
Pete *[laughs] How honest do you want us to be?*
CF *Very [laughs].*
Pete *Very honest, erm, I would say, my wife and I have always had a very, we've been married 38 years, erm, my brother-in-law used to describe us as sexual athletes.*
(Focus group with men with systemic sclerosis, UK)

Whenever I present my work or discuss it with healthcare professionals, they often ask me whether men prefer talking to male or female clinicians (see Chap. 9 for the answer!). I asked men with systemic sclerosis who they would prefer to talk to about sex, and there were mixed preferences with some preferring another man, others preferring women, but overall the majority took the approach that *"it don't matter if it's a male or female [doctor] just somebody that is knowledgeable of what's going on"* (Marshall, 51yrs, African American). These individual differences for physician gender preference were also apparent throughout the literature.

The below interaction from one of my focus groups with men with systemic sclerosis in the UK demonstrates these different preferences. Whilst Emil prefers a male clinician to avoid embarrassment in front of women, Karim suggests that a female clinician may be more understanding. Interestingly, Paul explains that although he would be happy with either a man or a woman, he may use different language to discuss issues related to sex and intimacy. Keeping his comments (below) in mind it becomes apparent that many of the men throughout my focus groups (as can be observed throughout the quotes used in this chapter) often medicalised or softened their language. Even in this interaction we can see that permission is subtly sought for him to tell me the language he would use with a male clinician. This suggests that traditional expectations for men to be respectful in front of women still prevail even in medical settings:

Paul	*If it's a male doctor, I'll be honest I will like come to the races, no problem. I'll talk to a male doctor. If it's a female doctor, I'll talk about it, but in a different way.*
CF	*And how would that be different?*
Paul	*It's just medical terminology. I'll go into amateur doctor mode. 'Ejaculation' or 'erection'. I will talk about it but a very sort of professional veil to it. Whereas, sorry, if a, er, bloke to bloke [laughs, hesitates] …*
CF	*It's okay.*
Paul	*… yeah, man to man.*
Emil	*Yeah.*
Karim	*Yes, yeah.*
Paul	*With a male doctor, it will be, 'well I can't get a hard-on Doc, I can't, can't perform' you know, and I'd get a bit more frank, with respect … Er, and, and it's easier, but I will talk about it to a female doctor. … But I prefer a male doctor, there lies my answer, I don't know what Emil and Karim think.*
Emil	*Yeah, it is something in that.*
Paul	*Is there something in that, is there, I wonder whether it is?*
Emil	*It is definitely an embarrassing thing.*
Paul	*Or is it me?*
Emil	*'Cause a man always feels like we have to be kind of macho-ish in front of a woman. So I think, I, I explain that, I feel embarrassed, I think you must be thinking I'm a bit worthless, but you know, I know it's silly but it, it is like that, you know, every man wants to feel like they're great in bed, or have a great experience but talking to a woman about it, you think, you know what I'm slacking, really bad and that, and you feel like, not like you've been judged but almost like you've been judged ….*
Karim	*You see I have no problem with that, talking to a woman doctor. I have no problem at all.*
Paul	*Different people, different strokes isn't it?*

Karim *I have no problem talking to women at all, in fact in some ways I'd prefer, because I think they'll probably understand it, as you say men would banter and joke around about it and whatever but I think they'll understand the problem.*
(Focus group with men with systemic sclerosis, UK)

Whilst we often concern ourselves with the gender preferences for healthcare professionals, interviews with young men (age 16–25) found that they not only generally preferred to talk about sex with a male GP, but it also seemed important to many of them that the healthcare professional was younger; they also highlighted wanting to be spoken to on equal terms without using jargon:

> *I wouldn't be able to talk to some old dude about it because that would just be creepy as. (James, 17yrs, Australia)* (Latreille et al., 2014)

Whilst men tended not to directly talk about erectile dysfunction to friends, they did seem to find it much easier to talk about times when the medication they were taking to improve blood flow to the extremities (e.g., sildenafil) caused unexpected erections. These situations perhaps lend themselves better to self-deprecating humour, enabling men to harness this to regain some control. However, it may also be that erections symbolise virility, which reinforce a masculine identity. Thus, male 'banter' around unexpected erections may be a form of humble bragging that their sexual prowess is not lost:

Pete *Yeah, my mates have had a right good laugh since I went onto sildenafil.*
James *Yeah, mine too [laughs], three times a day?*
Pete *I bet you hear it all as well don't you?*
James *Yeah. The only time I've an inappropriate erection was putting together a flat pack desk. Random …*
Frank *Ah, IKEA have got a lot to answer for then?*
James *Yeah, apparently it's because I was on my knees [laughs].*
(Focus group with men with systemic sclerosis, UK)

A suggestion from both my own focus groups and the wider literature was to provide spaces for men with similar sex and intimacy issues to discuss and resolve these together. The potential benefits of this on mental wellbeing were apparent throughout my focus group interactions, with men feeling less alone and sharing tips with each other. However, as illustrated by James (below), many men's ideal resolution would be to medically treat the physical issue (e.g., erectile dysfunction) rather than need to work through any resulting psychosocial issues:

> *I think it would be good to have a place where people can discuss their sexual issues. It will help them sort out their feelings by speaking out. They hear other people's opinions and realize that they share similar feelings. (sexual dysfunction associated with prostate cancer treatment, Japanese)* (Hayashi et al., 2023)

> *It's a male thing, they tend to be less emotional and more physiological, so I guess, you know, I think if you took a straw poll most blokes would say just give me a tablet if it's available. (James, 44yrs, systemic sclerosis, White British)*

Overall, this chapter has illustrated that across various cultures and conditions men will talk about sex and intimacy issues. Throughout the literature we can see that when directly asked or given permission to talk about sex, men have opened up in both one-to-one interviews and focus group settings with other men, and with both male and female researchers.

5.8 Summary

Sex and intimacy are highly valued by men in achieving positive quality of life with a long-term condition, and challenges to this can challenge their masculinity. The impact of long-term conditions on sex and intimacy is not limited to erectile dysfunction. Many other condition-specific physical symptoms can affect men's ability to fully engage in sexual activities in the way they want to, and broader impacts of illness on masculinity can translate to a lack of sexual confidence. Men worry about the impact of sex and intimacy issues on their relationships both physically in terms of the pleasure they are able to give their partner and emotional strains due to lost intimacy. Men with long-term conditions would like their clinical teams to ask about sex and intimacy as even though they are willing to talk this can be embarrassing for them to raise themselves. Whilst men would prefer the physical issues to be resolved through treatment or medication, failing this some men would value education and support, which may include their partners, or the opportunity to engage in problem-solving sessions with other men.

References

Alexis, O., & Worsley, A. J. (2018). A meta-synthesis of qualitative studies exploring men's sense of masculinity post-prostate cancer treatment. *Cancer Nursing, 41*(4), 298–310. https://doi.org/10.1097/NCC.0000000000000509

Bay, L. T., Graugaard, C., Nielsen, D. S., Möller, S., Ellingsen, T., & Giraldi, A. (2020). Sexual health and dysfunction in patients with rheumatoid arthritis: A cross-sectional single-center study. *Sexual Medicine, 8*(4), 615–630. https://doi.org/10.1016/J.ESXM.2020.07.004

Connell, R. W. (2005). *Masculinities* (2nd ed.). University of California Press.

Cooper, S., Leon, N., Namadingo, H., Bobrow, K., & Farmer, A. J. (2018). "My wife's mistrust. That's the saddest part of being a diabetic": A qualitative study of sexual well-being in men with Type 2 diabetes in sub-Saharan Africa. *PLOS ONE, 13*(9), e0202413. https://doi.org/10.1371/JOURNAL.PONE.0202413

Dyer, K., & das Nair, R. (2013). Why don't healthcare professionals talk about sex? A systematic review of recent qualitative studies conducted in the United Kingdom. *The Journal of Sexual Medicine, 10*(11), 2658–2670. https://doi.org/10.1111/J.1743-6109.2012.02856.X

Flurey, C., Pauling, J. D., Saketkoo, L. A., Denton, C. P., Galdas, P., Khanna, D., Williams, A., & Hughes, M. (2022). 'I turned in my man card': A qualitative study of the experiences, coping styles and support needs of men with systemic sclerosis. *Rheumatology, 62*(6), 2160–2167. https://doi.org/10.1093/RHEUMATOLOGY/KEAC585

Gerbild, H., Areskoug-Josefsson, K., Larsen, C. M., & Laursen, B. S. (2021). Acceptability of health professionals' address of sexuality and erectile dysfunction—A qualitative interview study with men in cardiac rehabilitation. *Sexual Medicine, 9*(3). https://doi.org/10.1016/J.ESXM.2021.100369

Hayashi, S., Sato, K., Oishi, F., Fukuda, H., Hayama, Y., & Ando, S. (2023). Care needs of Japanese men for sexual dysfunction associated with prostate cancer treatment. *Supportive Care in Cancer, 31*(7), 1–9. https://doi.org/10.1007/S00520-023-07837-W

Helland, Y., Garratt, A., Kjeken, I., Kvien, T., & Dagfinrud, H. (2013). Current practice and barriers to the management of sexual issues in rheumatology: Results of a survey of health professionals. *Scandinavian Journal of Rheumatology, 42*(1), 20–26. https://doi.org/10.3109/03009742.2012.709274

Jowett, A., Peel, E., & Shaw, R. L. (2011). Sex and diabetes: A thematic analysis of gay and bisexual men's accounts. *Journal of Health Psychology, 17*(3), 409–418. https://doi.org/10.1177/1359105311412838

Latreille, S., Collyer, A., & Temple-Smith, M. (2014). Finding a segue into sex: Young men's views on discussing sexual health with a GP. *Australian Family Physician, 43*(4), 217–221.

Letts, C., Tamlyn, K., & Byers, E. S. (2010). Exploring the impact of prostate cancer on men's sexual well-being. *Journal of Psychosocial Oncology, 28*(5), 490–510. https://doi.org/10.1080/07347332.2010.498457

Low, W. Y., Ng, C. J., Choo, W. Y., & Tan, H. M. (2009). How do men perceive erectile dysfunction and its treatment? A qualitative study on opinions of men. *The Aging Male, 9*(3), 175–180. https://doi.org/10.1080/13685530600914601

McDonagh, L. K., Nielsen, E. J., McDermott, D. T., Davies, N., & Morrison, T. G. (2017). "I want to feel like a full man": Conceptualizing gay, bisexual, and heterosexual men's sexual difficulties. *The Journal of Sex Research, 55*(6), 783–801. https://doi.org/10.1080/00224499.2017.1410519

Oliffe, J. (2005). Constructions of masculinity following prostatectomy-induced impotence. *Social Science & Medicine, 60*(10), 2249–2259. https://doi.org/10.1016/J.SOCSCIMED.2004.10.016

Östlund, G., Björk, M., Valtersson, E., & Sverker, A. (2015). Lived experiences of sex life difficulties in men and women with early RA—The Swedish TIRA project. *Musculoskeletal Care, 13*(4), 248–257. https://doi.org/10.1002/MSC.1105

Perez-Garcia, F. L., Röder, E., Pastoor, H., Bolt, J. M., van Exel, J., & Dolhain, E. M. R. J. (2021). It is not just about sex: Viewpoints of men with inflammatory arthritis on the overall impact of the disease on their sexual health Inflammatory arthritis. *RMD Open, 7.* https://doi.org/10.1136/rmdopen-2021-001821

Thongtang, P., Fongkaew, W., Sansiriphun, N., & Chaloumsuk, N. (2021). My thing is dead: Experience of dealing with diabetic erectile dysfunction of northern Thai men. *Pacific Rim International Journal of Nursing Research, 25*(2), 255–268.

CHAPTER 6

Mortality

"Oh my goodness me, I'm not invincible"

In writing this chapter it struck me how few papers I could find within the long-term conditions literature that focused on men's experiences or perceptions of facing death and dying. As you'll see throughout the chapter, mortality is addressed to some extent in the qualitative literature within a broader study remit focusing on experiences of living with life-limiting conditions (including my own in men with systemic sclerosis). However, I could only find one (Abbott et al., 2017) that specifically addressed death and dying as the primary aim of a study in men living with a long-term condition. Looking to the wider literature beyond long-term conditions, death doesn't often seem to be considered through a gendered lens. Yet, gender dynamics have been identified for those facing hospice death, with men struggling to reconcile potentially competing ideas of 'dying well' (a death that is pain free and allows time for acceptance, closure, and awareness) with preserving masculine ideals of not wanting to gradually become weaker and more dependent (Broom & Cavenagh, 2010).

Mortality was raised without prompting throughout my own focus groups with men with systemic sclerosis. Even for men who were well controlled with limited disease progression they were still aware of the shadow of living with a life-limiting condition. The awareness of their mortality was an unwelcome challenge to a masculine self-image of invincibility:

C. Flurey, *Talking Men's Health*,
https://doi.org/10.1007/978-3-031-62593-0_6

What's hit me is my mortality. That's what hit me, er, it's the first time someone has put a shot across my bows on my health and realising all of a sudden you wake up one morning, oh my goodness me, I'm not invincible. (Paul, 52yrs, systemic sclerosis, White British)

6.1 Threat of Mortality as a Wake-Up Call

At a population level, men are more likely to engage in lifestyle behaviours that act as risk factors for long-term conditions (e.g., smoking, drinking, fat and sugar consumption) (Lim et al., 2012). However, when faced with the threat of their mortality, some men experienced this as a wake-up call to look after their health:

I was angry. I was very angry because especially when I discovered how close I was to death. I was very angry. I was angry with myself after I discovered that what I thought I was doing right, eating right and so forth and this sort of thing was the cause of some of my issues with my health. (diabetes, African American) (Walker et al., 2022)

This newfound awareness of the need to look after their health meant having to depart from a construction of masculinity that dictates men don't look after their health. However, as discussed in Chap. 2, the action of taking responsibility for their health can align with masculine ideals of control and self-reliance. Thus, taking action to look after their health whether through diet and exercise, or through advocating for their need to rest or not over-exert themselves, may be one way they can regain some control over their lives and their health:

I think [the diagnosis of cancer] really emphasized that for me the fact that I had vulnerabilities of this nature. That I needed to stay focused a little more on my health in terms of eating properly and losing some weight and getting some more exercise, and that sort of thing. (P-1, breast cancer, USA) (Potter et al., 2023)

6.2 Medical Management of Mortality

For men who were living with a life-limiting condition but not yet facing end of life, it was important to them that their treatment was as effective as possible to prevent the progression or spread of disease. Many of these men had developed a strong understanding of the different treatment options through discussions with their medical team and their own research. They were often acutely aware of the severity of their condition and the potential consequences of leaving it unmanaged. John describes the approach to his treatment regime of using early aggressive treatment to prevent the progression of systemic sclerosis, demonstrating his understanding of the clinical decision-making:

John *Yeah, and yet hopefully they can keep it in the first stage, I mean that certainly I think seems to be the goal, they seem to really try to aggressively keep it in the first stage, and not let it move.*
CF *Is that a worry for most of you, it spreading to internal organs?*
Scott *Oh yeah.*
John *Certainly your, your goose is kinda cooked at that point, in a way, I mean you can survive and they can treat each thing as it comes along but yeah, you're, it's going to do some damage, it's going to leave a mark once it progresses.*
(Focus group with men with systemic sclerosis, USA)

For those who were facing end of life, the choice between accepting life-prolonging treatment versus preserving their quality of life was an individual one. Men balanced the pros and cons of each considering both the quality and length of their lives. Some men discussed this with family and friends to help make a decision. Whilst some sought out as much information as possible from various sources, others preferred to rely on their oncologist or oncology nurse. Previous experiences of cancer treatments (their own or someone close to them) also contributed to their decision-making, with negative experiences reinforcing fears and worries. Men talked about prolonging life to spend more time with friends and family, to reach future personal 'milestones' such as seeing a child or grandchild graduate, to spend more time on their hobbies, or to go back to work (Doveson et al., 2020).

In terms of discussing their mortality with their clinical team, this often seemed to be approached from a medical rather than psychological perspective. Some men told stories of their doctors being blunt with them about their prognosis or being visibly uncomfortable. One clinician told me he gets a 'heart sink' when diagnosing men with systemic sclerosis due to the mortality rate (twice as high in men as in women), which may explain the doctor's reaction that John describes:

John *Yeah that's kind of funny, the doctor that diagnosed me back in January of this year, with scleroderma, her first comment. She just kind of looked at me, wouldn't, didn't even make eye contact with me, looked down at my hands and, and, er, she said, 'you know I had a guy in here just, we caught it just at this stage with him, he didn't make it through the year'.*
Jim *Oh my goodness.*
John *It just kind of framed it right away, she said, 'yeah, this is serious'. (Focus group with men with systemic sclerosis, USA)*

Some men had experienced conversations about resuscitation, with mixed responses on whether these were handled sensitively. Either way, many men highlighted the lack of discussion around the emotional side of death. There seemed to be a distinct lack of opportunity to talk about death beyond the practical side of medical management:

> *Doctors say a lot when you're diagnosed—you won't be able to walk, you'll have to go into a wheelchair—then they suddenly stop when you come to death. It's odd really because they're leading you to the door of the conversation but they're keeping it closed which makes it more scary really. (R9, 25yrs, Duchenne muscular dystrophy, Asian British)* (Abbott et al., 2017)

The best time to talk about death will be different for everyone, so it would be reasonable for clinicians to worry about raising this at a time that causes unnecessary upset. However, most men report being unlikely to bring this up themselves but were happy to be asked even if they chose not to discuss it at that time. For clinicians working with people with life-limiting conditions, the following quote is such an incredibly powerful and important point, highlighting the importance of clinician communication and treating the whole person:

> *He asks about my life and that's the difference and it means you don't mind talking about anything really. If you can talk about how you live then you can talk about dying. It's difficult to talk about your death to someone who may not be that interested in your life. (R11, 21yrs, Duchenne muscular dystrophy, White British)* (Abbott et al., 2017)

6.3 Death and Taxes: Protector and Provider Responsibilities

The value of the protector and provider role to many men was discussed in Chap. 2, and men seem to feel the weight of these responsibilities even when faced with their mortality. Many men living with a life-limiting condition discussed worries about their families coping financially after their death and took steps to help their families prepare to manage without them. For example, American citizens are responsible for filing tax returns, and Scott discusses how he recently taught his wife how to do this:

> *This year when we did taxes, I normally always do the taxes and then I review it with my wife when it's done and we both sign the documents, so this year we actually both did the taxes. […] I would have continued to just do the taxes myself but I figured she better know how to do this. And in a lot of other areas it's been like that where I've involved her a lot more and, and things like that, financial things like that, because I, I just don't really know what the future's like. (Scott, 43yrs, systemic sclerosis, White American)*

Men discussed taking actions to make things easier for their families after their death such as getting legal documents in order and making plans for their funerals (Doveson et al., 2020). Younger men also talked about wanting to put their affairs in order but felt they would need support and weren't sure who they could ask for help. Although they often hadn't spoken to anyone about it, for many men music choices for their funerals mattered to them (Abbott et al., 2017). Men also worried about the emotional impact on their loved ones and often described feeling a responsibility to protect them from the full picture. They worried about how others would cope emotionally when they were no longer there:

> *The biggest thing I worry about is what happens to everyone else. It sounds weird but it's like if you die you're letting them down or something. I worry that they will be upset. (R3, 30yrs, Duchenne muscular dystrophy, White British)* (Abbott et al., 2017)

6.4 Longing for a Life That May Not Be Lived

Men talked about death in terms of a life they may be missing out on, and reflected on what they may or may not live to see and experience. This grief for a potentially lost life seemed to be an emotional trigger for many men, rather than specific symptoms or fear of death itself:

> *There's the odd occasion [coughs] when your body is so weak that you do get emotional but usually for me, certainly last year with the, say, radiotherapy and other people call it their dark days, it's not that you feel sorry for yourself, it's the things that possibly you're not gonna to be able to do again. You're not gonna to be able to see Star Wars 28 in five years' time. It's the silly things. I might not be able to go back to my home-town and things, and that's what gets you, certainly for me. Otherwise, no, you can't dwell on it. I've got to this age, fine. (Frank, 64yrs, systemic sclerosis, White British)*

Most poignantly, men discussed a life they had pictured with their children or grandchildren, which they worried they may no longer be able to fulfil. Within the focus groups these were the topics that brought the men to tears as they listened to each other's dreams for a future with their families and reflected on their own:

> *I think about it in terms of what I will or maybe not be able to do with my daughter that before I had her, before I got sick I was like, oh when I have a child, like these are the types of things I want to do with them. (Scott, 43yrs, systemic sclerosis, White American)*

> *You say you want your grandchildren to remember you, I want to see my grandchildren. (Paul, 52yrs, systemic sclerosis, White British)*

6.5 Living with an Uncertain Timeline

Living with a life-limiting condition can mean living with the sword of Damocles hanging over their head. For those living with cancer, having their cancer staged, and being given a prognosis could give them a clearer sense of their future. However, this still left an element of uncertainty around how their disease may progress and what the future will hold. Oscar who was given a 70% chance of survival uses humour to express this fear of 'what if':

> *[I've] been to the Casino with a lot worse (laughing) odds than that, um, but at the same time you [...] start thinking what happens if... you know supposing I don't come out of this? (Oscar, late 50s, head/neck cancer, Canada)* (Wenger, 2013)

Although they didn't know when it would come, the awareness of death looming in their future gave men an appreciation of the fragility of life and their own mortality. For some men this provoked a desire to live life to the fullest as if every day was their last. For example, Mark, who had gone through a period he wasn't sure he would survive, talks about the importance to him of living without regrets:

> *There was a little bit when, erm, it wasn't absolutely [laughs] certain I was going to [live], and, erm, yeah, so you're left with, well you could be there again, don't have anything left that you didn't, that you wish you hadn't done this time, go and do it [laughs] if you possibly can. (Mark, systemic sclerosis, White British)*

However, for some men the uncertain timeline on their mortality left them questioning how best to spend their time. There was a balance to be struck between living life to the full for short-term gains versus saving resources for a potential future. Men were aware there may not be a future of their own to plan for, but still felt the provider responsibility to consider stability for their family or their own potential future. Some men questioned the value of putting time and effort into long-term goals with the uncertainty over whether they would live to see the benefits:

Paul	*I don't know how to play it. Do you go reckless and open yourself to the world and live your life 10,000 percent, do you find a middle ground, pitch it in the middle ...*
Karim	*You do what you can.*
Paul	*You vaguely do anyway, you value life more if you experience it. (Focus group with men with systemic sclerosis, UK)*

> *[D]o I really want to start big things like going to school for the next four years or six years or for even thinking about a PhD because am I even going to be around? A lot of the guys we've seen just go from healthy with Barth to just boof! (Barth syndrome, USA)* (Mazar & Moorman, 2021)

6.6 Emotional Impact of Mortality

Despite a popular social narrative that men don't talk in ways that show weakness or vulnerability, in both my own studies and throughout the literature many men explicitly discussed the emotional impact of facing their mortality. Men openly expressed worries and fears about their disease progressing or spreading, and the impact of this on the length and quality of their lives:

> *I've been investigated for scleroderma in the heart 'cause my heart was pumping so hard my chest, my lungs were hurting so much I was scared, and oh my word, what's going on, so I've spent the last six months with them investigating my heart and everything, I think, oh please I don't want scleroderma in the heart 'cause it will just fail, so I've been scared out of my life. (Emil, 37yrs, systemic sclerosis, Black British)*

Some men talked openly about the distress that they experienced in mourning for the life they may not get to live. Karim explains that although he is focused on making the most of the life he has left, he still cries himself to sleep over the thought of losing out on time with family, or his grandchildren growing up without knowing him:

> *For the first three months I used to cry every night, every night I used to cry. [...] I want to look after my grandchildren, I want my grandchildren to remember me, you know, and, and all this goes through your mind. I still get that, every so often, maybe once a week, once a month, once every three months. You know, but and then I cry myself to sleep. (Karim, systemic sclerosis, British Asian)* (Flurey et al., 2022)

Some men discussed worries and fears around the process of dying. Many of these fears seemed to stem from the uncertainty of what it would be like to die. They worried about whether they would be in pain or suffer. Some wondered about which part of their condition would ultimately cause their death. Some had experienced family members dying without their pain being managed and were afraid of the same fate, others had formed ideas through the media, and some were simply scared of the unknown (Doveson et al., 2020). Some discussed suicide and euthanasia as a way of maintaining an element of control and allowing them to die without pain. Overall, many men with life-limiting conditions wanted to know what would happen at the point of dying :

It's specific things you want to know about what is the last stage going to look like? Are you going to be gasping for breath and in pain and all sorts of horrible things? Or will it be potentially peaceful? (R1, 34yrs, Duchenne muscular dystrophy, White British) (Abbott et al., 2017)

As Katheryn Mannix discusses in her TEDx talk, *"What happens as we die"* (which I would thoroughly recommend to anyone who may one day die), whilst death can be full of uncertainty and fear there are commonalities across end of life death that could be explained to patients and their families to ease some of this fear of the unknown (Mannix, 2022).

Some men also considered the uncertainty of what comes after death. Those who had a faith seemed to take comfort in the belief of an afterlife. A meta-synthesis of qualitative studies in prostate cancer found Black British, African American, and Latin American men frequently spoke of spirituality, generally in Christian terms, and turned to their beliefs to help them cope (Rivas et al., 2016). Those without a faith took a more pragmatic approach, with some taking comfort in the belief that there is nothing to worry about coming next, life just stops. One of my focus groups with American men included strongly held views on both sides, with the discussion needing to be moved on to avoid an argument. Hank seemed frustrated at the beliefs of those who sought comfort in their faith, and it's possible his atheist views may have been strengthened with the feeling of unfairness of living with a life-limiting condition:

Hank	*I don't know how many people here believe in God, but I don't, that's a bunch of bullshit.*
Jacob	*I believe in God.*
Wade	*I believe very strongly.*
Hank	*You'll get a rude awakening, 'cause when it's over, it's over. (Focus group with men with systemic sclerosis, USA)*

Social support will be discussed further in Chap. 9, but it is worth noting here that despite the emotional toll that the worry and fear of death was taking, many men didn't feel able to discuss this with their families:

When you're talking about what will happen when you're at death's door, that's kind of hard to talk about with my mum, dad, sister and that. (R7, 27yrs, Duchenne muscular dystrophy, White British) (Abbott et al., 2017)

6.7 Choosing Avoidance

Whilst some men highlighted the value of opening-up about their emotions surrounding end of life, others found that this caused them to focus on something they would rather not think about. Some men were reluctant to be reminded of the fear and vulnerability associated with facing death and couldn't see any value in talking to others about something they would find painful to focus on:

> *...I ignore that completely because I think it is crazy ... I have enough to work on with my own disease and should I then need to talk to others with the same disease ... they are talking about how bad they are feeling in that case I will feel even more ill... (I4, advanced prostate cancer, Sweden)* (Jonsson et al., 2009)

Some men explained that being put into situations that made them think about their condition caused them to focus and reflect on their mortality, which affected their mental wellbeing and ability to cope. Thus, some men coped by choosing to purposefully avoid things that would act as an unwelcome reminder:

> *When I'm asked questions or I read a newspaper article about cancer, it [thoughts about death] all comes back and then I get anxious and have problems with sleeping. (IP6, prostate cancer, Sweden)* (Wennick et al., 2017)

Others didn't so much shy away from the discussion of death completely but discussed it in a detached and pragmatic or even flippant way. There is perhaps an element of shared group bravado in the following exchange as quotes from the same participants throughout this chapter do indicate that at times they have worried about death or disease progression. The philosophy of only worrying about the things you can control is a useful mantra as a coping strategy but may not always be as easy in practice. However, this idealised approach perhaps helps reconcile a masculine need for control with the uncertain nature of death and dying through focusing on the things that are within control such as focusing on living life to the full:

Pete *We're all going to croak one day.*
James *Death and taxes, death and taxes. ... We're all going to die of something aren't we?*

Pete *Exactly, get on and live your life, so that's what we do. Erm, my family has a nasty habit of dropping dead quite young anyway [laughs]. [...] No, get out there and do your stuff, that's my philosophy. [...]*

Frank *If it's not definite then there's no point in even thinking about it to be honest.*

Pete *Only worry about the things you can impact, don't worry about other stuff [laughs].*

Frank *The things that you can impact, I've always been of the philosophy that if you want, wanna do something do it before it's too late, er, 'cause you never know what's round the corner, but by God the last four years have really enhanced that thought.*
(Focus group with men with systemic sclerosis, UK)

6.8 Gallows Humour

Gallows humour treats serious, frightening, or painful subject matter in a light or satirical way. If you search the literature for gallows humour, the majority of papers focus on healthcare professionals or emergency service workers use of this humour to cope with the experiences of death and trauma they encounter in their working lives. The literature seems quite divided on whether gallows humour is acceptable amongst professionals or not. Some acknowledge it as a protective coping strategy that is acceptable as long as it is kept 'behind the scenes' away from the public's ears (Watson, 2011). Whilst others see gallows humour from professionals as deprecating and insulting to those under their care or protection (Piemonte, 2015). In terms of patient and healthcare professional interaction, humour is seen as beneficial to build rapport, yet healthcare professionals are cautioned against the use of humour in relation to tragedy or sensitive topics. However, men discussed valuing clinicians who *"tune into your sense of humour straight away"* (Frank).

Men in my own studies and throughout the literature used gallows humour as a way of tackling the serious, frightening, and painful matter of their own deaths. Humour was often used as a way of expressing difficult sentiments, which may be an attempt to make these topics easier on the interviewer rather than simply a self-protective coping strategy. Roy, who had a short time left to live, describes a philosophical consideration of the afterlife, which he goes on to lighten with humour perhaps to rebalance the interview to a more upbeat tone:

> *I say to family I've got a lot of things to tell Mum and Dad, and my two brothers and my sisters when I get there [heaven] … of course the general knowledge is that's not possible, but I say it must be a good place. I've never heard of anybody coming back. (Roy, advanced prostate cancer Anglo-Australian)* (Oliffe, 2006)

Men talked about the value of having people to talk to who used humour rather than shying away from the topic of death. Younger men with Duchenne muscular dystrophy generally didn't speak to friends who did not have this condition about death as they felt the conversation was closed down. However, they valued speaking to others with the same condition as they felt able to talk to them about end of life, and use humour in a way that made them feel understood:

> *I always think it's easier to talk to lads with MD because they're in the same boat and they understand. There's always dark humour and stuff. Yeah, we do talk about ourselves and stuff like end of life. (R3, 30yrs, Duchenne muscular dystrophy, White British)* (Abbott et al., 2017)

By contrast, men with systemic sclerosis had generally not met another man with their condition prior to taking part in the focus groups, so were unable to comment on the value of shared understandings. However, for some who spoke to their friends about their condition they were often met with dark humour, which they appreciated. Whilst the interaction may at the most surface-level interpretation seem as if Frank's friends are uncaring, he and other men generally understood responses such as these as an expression of how much their friends care about them—that they needed to make light of the situation to help with their own discomfort. Frank points out this is *"the way blokes deal with it"*, with gallows humour perhaps aligning to masculine ideals of stoicism and strength, men laugh in the face of death:

Frank *One of my oldest friends, he said, 'Frank, you're going, having this operation tomorrow?' 'Yeah', 'and it's okay, isn't it?' 'Yeah, it's fine, it's only a minor one'. He says, 'look, if you don't make it can I have your new drill?' [laughing], and then all the others chipped in, 'oh, hang on about, blah, blah'. Now when I tell the women that, they're horrified but that's just the way blokes deal with it. […] Gallows humour, or battlefield humour as they called it in the army apparently, and I love that, I absolutely love that. I've got no problem with it at all.*

CF *And is that quite a male way of coping, to make light of things?*

Frank *I think so, I think so, 'cause like I say most women I've told have been horrified at that, 'how do you cope, you can't say that?' You know, about the tools … and he's still asking for them now [laughs] (Focus group with men with systemic sclerosis, UK)*

One man (below) with prostate cancer explains that although he can see the dark humour in a situation it's not always easy to see the funny side. This may perhaps serve as a caution that whilst men may choose to use gallows humour to help express themselves it may not always be welcome to engage in without permission:

> *One day when I checked the Internet for complementary medicine … the number for the crematory came up (laughter). I saw the humour in it, but it is not always easy to take it humorously. (prostate cancer, Norway)* (Ervik & Asplund, 2012)

There may also be a cultural element to the use of dark humour in the face of death with this being commonly identified in studies with participants from Northwest Europe or Australia. In my systemic sclerosis focus groups, dark humour was apparent in my UK but not my USA groups. This cultural discomfort with dark humour was further highlighted by an American co-author who expressed uncertainty with my use of the following quote to introduce a theme of dark humour in the resulting paper. Tim's implication here is that he may not be alive to see the bananas ripen:

> *Like that film [The second best exotic marigold hotel] where she said, you know Maggie Smith said I've stopped buying green bananas [laughs]. (Tim, systemic sclerosis, White British)* (Flurey et al., 2022)

6.9 Summary

For men with life-limiting long-term conditions, mortality is a constant background worry. The responsibility to take on a protector and provider role in the family prevails in the face of mortality with many men taking steps to ensure their families are able to cope when they are no longer around. Men grieve the loss of their potential life and especially mourn the things they anticipated being able to do with children or grandchildren. Living with an uncertain timeline can challenge masculine ideals of control. Some deal with this by regaining control through living life to the full, whilst others try to find a balance with the provider responsibility to save and plan for a future they may not be part of. Some men use gallows humour to talk about death, which can help them open up about their fears in a way they may perceive as more comfortable to the person they are talking to. These men often value others who will understand and join in with this humour. However, despite the social narrative that men don't cry, some men will talk candidly about their emotions and did openly cry with each other in my focus groups. Clinicians should talk to men about the emotional as well as medical side of death (or signpost to appropriate support) and help to demystify the dying process.

References

Abbott, D., Prescott, H., Forbes, K., Fraser, J., & Majumdar, A. (2017). Men with Duchenne muscular dystrophy and end of life planning. *Neuromuscular Disorders, 27*(1), 38–44.

Broom, A., & Cavenagh, J. (2010). Masculinity, moralities and being cared for: An exploration of experiences of living and dying in a hospice. *Social Science & Medicine, 71*(5), 869–876. https://doi.org/10.1016/J.SOCSCIMED.2010.05.026

Doveson, S., Holm, M., Axelsson, L., Fransson, P., & Wennman-Larsen, A. (2020). Facing life-prolonging treatment: The perspectives of men with advanced metastatic prostate cancer—An interview study. *European Journal of Oncology Nursing, 49*. https://doi.org/10.1016/j.ejon.2020.101859

Ervik, B., & Asplund, K. (2012). Dealing with a troublesome body: A qualitative interview study of men's experiences living with prostate cancer treated with endocrine therapy. *European Journal of Oncology Nursing, 16*(2), 103–108. https://doi.org/10.1016/J.EJON.2011.04.005

Flurey, C., Pauling, J. D., Saketkoo, L. A., Denton, C. P., Galdas, P., Khanna, D., Williams, A., & Hughes, M. (2022). 'I turned in my man card': A qualitative study of the experiences, coping styles and support needs of men with systemic sclerosis. *Rheumatology, 62*(6), 2160–2167. https://doi.org/10.1093/RHEUMATOLOGY/KEAC585

Jonsson, A., Aus, G., & Bertero, C. (2009). Men's experience of their life situation when diagnosed with advanced prostate cancer. *European Journal of Oncology Nursing, 13*, 268–273.

Lim, S. S., Vos, T., Flaxman, A. D., Danaei, G., Shibuya, K., Adair-Rohani, H., AlMazroa, M. A., Amann, M., Anderson, H. R., & Andrews, K. G. (2012). A comparative risk assessment of burden of disease and injury attributable to 67 risk factors and risk factor clusters in 21 regions, 1990–2010: A systematic analysis for the Global Burden of Disease Study 2010. *The Lancet, 380*(9859), 2224–2260.

Mannix, K. (2022, November). *What happens as we die?* TEDx.

Mazar, I., & Moorman, S. M. (2021). "I want that life a lot…how on earth do I get that?" Examining challenges for men with Barth Syndrome in their transitions to adulthood. *Journal of Patient Experience, 8*. https://doi.org/10.1177/23743735211060783

Oliffe, J. (2006). Embodied masculinity and androgen deprivation therapy. *Sociology of Health & Illness, 28*(4), 410–432. https://doi.org/10.1111/J.1467-9566.2006.00499.X

Piemonte, N. M. (2015). Last laughs: Gallows humor and medical education. *Journal of Medical Humanities, 36*(4), 375–390. https://doi.org/10.1007/S10912-015-9338-4

Potter, A. M., Bentz, B., Crue, L., Leiby, S., Bashi, S., Maguire, K., Meyers, J., & Mieczkowski, K. (2023). Men's lived experiences of breast cancer and changes in occupation. *Occupational Therapy International.* https://doi.org/10.1155/2023/9641922

Rivas, C., Matheson, L., Nayoan, J., Glaser, A., Gavin, A., Wright, P., Wagland, R., & Watson, E. (2016). Ethnicity and the prostate cancer experience: A qualitative metasynthesis. In *Psycho-Oncology* (Vol. 25, Issue 10, pp. 1147–1156). https://doi.org/10.1002/pon.4222

Walker, A. Q., Blake, C. E., Moore, J. B., Wilcox, S., DuBois, K., Watkins, W., & K. (2022). Experiences of midlife and older African American men living with type 2 diabetes. *Ethnicity & Health, 27*(6), 1256–1270. https://doi.org/10.1080/13557858.2021.1910206

Watson, K. (2011). Gallows humor in medicine. *Hastings Center Report, 41*(5), 37–45.

Wenger, L., & Oliffe, J. (2013). Men managing cancer: A gender analysis. *Sociology of Health & Illness, 36*(1), 108–122. https://doi.org/10.1111/1467-9566.12045

Wennick, A., Jönsson, A. K., Bratt, O., & Stenzelius, K. (2017). Everyday life after a radical prostatectomy—A qualitative study of men under 65 years of age. *European Journal of Oncology Nursing, 30*, 107–112. https://doi.org/10.1016/J.EJON.2017.08.008

CHAPTER 7

Coping and Self-management

"You've got take your own case and you gotta take it on like it's a job"

Chapter 2 covered the many ways that living with a long-term condition can affect masculine ideals such as strength, stoicism, and self-reliance, and how this can challenge their sense of power and control over their lives. Many of the coping strategies that I will discuss in the current chapter seem to provide a way of reclaiming some of this lost control. It seems important to men to find ways of managing their condition that puts them in the driver's seat. For some, this may mean controlling as much of their lives as possible to put their health first. For others, this can be making a deliberate decision not to let their condition hold them back, although there may be painful consequences. As the young man below explains, enabling men to make their own decisions about managing their condition can be empowering. Finding ways to reclaim power and control may be important for protecting masculine status:

> *They think I'm a bit more fragile than I am. Making decisions about the support I get is really important. It gives me more power and makes me feel … yeah. But I am in control, it is my—I mean it's my life, so. (Duchenne muscular dystrophy, UK)* (Abbott et al., 2016)

C. Flurey, *Talking Men's Health*,
https://doi.org/10.1007/978-3-031-62593-0_7

7.1 Managing the Physical Condition

Men can often be assumed to be poor at looking after their health and wellbeing. However, this isn't necessarily the case. In fact, when faced with a threat to their health men often seem to reclaim control of their condition through taking responsibility for looking after their bodies. In addition to specific symptom management, men throughout the literature often mention a general focus on lifestyle health behaviours (such as diet, exercise, reduced alcohol consumption) to minimise the impact of their condition. This shift to what Prof Steve Robertson terms a 'should care' approach to their health has been noted in men's responses to experiencing an acute cardiac event (Robertson et al., 2010). Thus, it seems that a change in health status, whether acute or chronic, can re-orient men's attention towards their health.

Men with long-term conditions seem to be no less informed than women about the various ways to self-manage their physical symptoms and often shared tips with each other in the focus groups. For example, men with systemic sclerosis described regularly using moisturiser to stay on top of their dry skin and gave each other tips on where to buy the best heated gloves to control the extreme cold felt in their fingers. Far from being unbothered about their health, for many men mastering control over symptom management and being able to share their knowledge with others seemed to be a matter of pride. Below, a man with diabetes describes how he followed the self-management guidance to the point his diabetes is controlled without medication. He talks about his 'numbers' going down, which was also commonly seen in my own studies with men being aware of their 'numbers' in relation to inflammatory markers. It's worth considering that gamification (the application of typical elements of game playing [e.g., point scoring, competition with self or others, rules of play] to encourage engagement) could be an effective way of supporting men to stay on track with self-management, as many seem motivated by the 'achievement' of seeing their biomarkers improve:

> *I'm off [medication]. I did the exercise and lost weight, and so my numbers went back down by going through the education process and doing whatever they said. I got away from diabetes. I'm not … I'm not diabetic no more. (type 2 diabetes, African American)* (Walker et al., 2022)

Men often describe taking responsibility for their health through pacing themselves and acknowledging their limitations. They made efforts to listen to their bodies and stop before they overdid things. This could be seen as a departure from masculinity as it rejects a 'no pain no gain' approach or pushing themselves to their limits. However, there is masculine value in being able to exert self-control, and many men with long-term conditions express the benefits of pacing themselves. George describes this as *'overcoming'* indicating a reclaiming of control through mastering this form of self-management. It's worth noting again that this strategy of timing himself could also be seen as a form of gamifying self-management:

> *I time myself, you know, sort of like an hour, and if I've been an hour, I stop, no matter what I hadn't done and then that way around I find I can get more hours in in the week, whereas if you went on that extra hour, you're wiped for the next day, so that's how I overcome it. (George, 74yrs, systemic sclerosis, White British)*

In masculine environments, such as the workplace or in friendship groups, men often have to advocate for themselves to put their health first. In Chap. 2 I discussed how men may have to negotiate protecting their health with maintaining their masculine status. In the work environment, some dealt with this through exerting their authority in leadership roles to delegate physical tasks to others. James is self-employed and explains how he had to tell a client he was unable to continue working for the day. He explains he did the *'sensible thing'*, thus centring masculine values of taking responsibility:

> *I had to stop, I said to my client, 'I'm sorry I've got to go back' and apparently I looked like a corpse, so he said, 'yeah come back next week' [laughs]. I did the sensible thing I went home, I laid down, and I got up in the evening and I felt, you know, a thousand times better, just very tired. (James, 44yrs, systemic sclerosis, White British)* (Flurey et al., 2022)

Similarly to findings in women, many men described trying anything they could to minimise the impact of their condition. Beyond trying all the self-management recommendations from their clinical teams, men also tried alternative therapies or tips from other patients such as cutting out certain foods (e.g., some people with rheumatoid arthritis suggest that tomatoes aggravate their symptoms). Trying things beyond management recommended by their clinical team was for some men another way of reclaiming some control over their condition, giving them hope, and a feeling of being proactive:

> *[F]ood supplements, herbs, various herbal supplements ... you think they gonna help cure your cancer. ... you feel that there's some hope in there ... you feel that that can boost your immune system, and also that some of those will have a cancer-killing effect. ... [I] felt better ... had some sort of control over ... treatment and ... outcomes. (cancer, Australian)* (Klafke et al., 2014)

7.2 Retaining Autonomy Within a Medical Model

A few years ago, the phrase "please don't confuse your Google search with my medical degree" started to spread through social media in response to the growing culture of patients researching their symptoms online prior to consultations. In response to this, the patient communities responded with variations of the phrase "please don't confuse your medical degree with my life" (Ireland, 2019). It's important to remember that individuals have their own expertise, different experiences, different needs, and different priorities. For those with long-term conditions they've often had many years of living with and managing their condition and know what works best for them on a day-to-day basis. Despite pithy social media phrases, it is important to acknowledge that a broad shift towards shared decision-making in healthcare (patients and clinicians working together to make treatment decisions) has been a positive step towards ensuring these individual differences are taken into consideration and patients are empowered and supported to make the best decisions for themselves.

The way men talked about their clinical teams varied, which will be explored further in Chap. 9. Whilst some placed more trust or reverence in their clinicians than others, the men broadly accepted that their clinical team held the expertise in treating their conditions. However, for many men it was still important to retain their autonomy within the medical model of treatment management. Some men discussed making changes to their treatment regime either with or without their clinician's knowledge. For some this could be skipping doses or changing the days of their medication to avoid side effects coinciding with an upcoming event, or to enable them to drink alcohol. Whilst for others (e.g., David) this could be increasing the dose to manage a flare of their condition:

Between you and me, yeah. Instead of taking like two sulfasalazine, I might ... for a couple of days, I know I won't ... I might take three. And er three in the morning, still take two at night or whatever and just up the dose a wee bit until it calms down. (David, 58yrs, rheumatoid arthritis, White British)

Men discussed the importance of making their own decisions in weighing up impact of treatment on their quality of life. For example, some men with cancer rejected pain medication, medical interventions (e.g., feeding tube), or invasive treatment that interfered with their ability to continue with valued activities, or to prioritise quality over length of life (Wenger & Oliffe, 2013). This may sometimes feel at odds with medical management, which often prioritises treatment with psychological impact considered second. However, patient priorities don't always align with those of healthcare professionals, and this demonstrates the importance of treating the whole patient not just the physical symptoms.

Men also discussed the need to take an active role in advocating for themselves in the medical system. Some talked about proactively asking their clinicians about medication they'd heard about through other patients, research journals, or the media. The interaction below acknowledges the importance of taking control of their own health and not simply waiting for the medical team to ask, which can be particularly important with a condition like systemic sclerosis where symptoms can vary widely from patient to patient:

Ted *Because everybody's different, you may not be having the same troubles I do.*

Jorge *Exactly.*

Travis *You've definitely got to be proactive, everybody's different, you've got take your own case and you gotta take it on like it's a job.*
(Focus group with men with systemic sclerosis, USA) (Flurey et al., 2022)

7.3 Destructive Behaviours or Calculated Risks?

Research suggests that men and boys are more likely to engage in risk-taking behaviours than women, with risk factors being responsible for more male than female deaths on a global scale (Lim et al., 2012). Thus, when it comes to managing a long-term condition, we might reasonably expect men to take more risks with their health. However, risk-taking behaviours in response to long-term conditions may not always be due to a reckless disregard for their health. Many men talked about pushing themselves to continue with a task beyond the point they were comfortable or may experience consequences the next day. However, as discussed in the previous section retaining autonomy can be important to men in coping with a long-term condition. Thus, what might be thought of as 'overdoing it' was often a conscious decision having weighed up the pros and cons and concluding, it's worth it:

Pete *So, my new boy's toy arrived [log splitter] and it had to be put together really, and I was outside doing it, erm, and I, wear kind of nice thin gloves, it, it protects you from getting dirty hands but also it gives you that little bit of insulation and I was out there, and I'm not kidding, my hands were hanging off in the cold. I thought I'm not going to give up putting this together and I kept going until it got dark and I couldn't work on it anymore because it was too dark to see. But when I came in, I was chilled completely to the core even though I was well wrapped up …*

James *Yeah, a hot bath, when it gets in your hands, it gets to the bones doesn't it?*

Pete *Erm, it had got that bad, erm, and it had gone right into me, erm, and when I went to bed that night and this is many hours later and I didn't go to bed until about 11:30, erm, I was cold all night in bed, and couldn't sleep properly. So maybe I should be listening to my body, but I'm refusing to on the basis of I'm not giving in.*

CF *So did you regret that, or was it worth it?*

Pete *It was worth it. It's like when you go skiing, it was worth it, even though sometimes you're coming off the slopes and you're almost crying with the pain if you've got really cold, you still want to do it, because there'll come a time when I really can't do it.*
(Focus group with men with systemic sclerosis, UK)

When weighing up the pros and cons of risk-taking behaviours, men may not always come to the same conclusion that would be welcomed by their clinical team. Some men discussed self-medicating with alcohol or recreational drugs. They were often aware of the negative effects of these drugs but prioritised the short-term benefits of symptom control. This was often as a form of pain relief, but as Jacob (below) explains cannabis was also used to improve appetite, which can be impacted by systemic sclerosis. As systemic sclerosis is a condition that can affect the lungs, clinicians have been particularly surprised to hear that men with systemic sclerosis would choose smoking cannabis to control their symptoms. This flags the importance of understanding men's decision-making in adopting risk-taking behaviours. Chastising or discouraging men from cannabis use is likely to only lead to the behaviour not being disclosed to clinicians. Thus, it may be more effective to discuss alternative methods for cannabis use to reduce the impact on the lungs, or whether any symptoms could be better controlled with medical management:

Jacob	*I smoke marijuana, junk, with my brother. I have two puffs, I ate up the whole damn house [laughs]. She [his wife] was up in that kitchen all damn night. I'm having them if they make me eat, I know how to eat. I go smoke it in the back yard and I'm going right in the house and get my table set up [laughing]. It helps.*
CF	*So does weed help with your symptoms?*
Jacob	*It helps me sleep.*
CF	*It helps you sleep.*
Jacob	*Yeah, it's good.*
CF	*Does it help with the pain?*
Jacob	*Yeah, yeah.*
Hank	*It helps somewhat with the pain, they got really good weed now.*
Jacob	*It takes your mind off, you know, it takes you mind off, it might be hurting you but after you get that high that damn, that pain gone. Now I when I dried out, the pain right back.*
	(Focus group with men with systemic sclerosis, USA)

Whilst some men seem to be making an informed decision to engage in risk-taking behaviours in relation to their long-term condition, for others it can be due to seeing no other options. Steve describes *'punishing'* himself with physical activity as a way of dealing with his emotions in response to living with rheumatoid arthritis. This level of high impact activity has the potential to be causing irreversible future joint damage, which he acknowledges (*"I'm going to pay for it in the long run"*). Thus, men may resort to risk-taking behaviours that can cause themselves damage when they see no other option. This makes it crucial that appropriate support is developed (see Chap. 9) to enable men to identify and adopt healthy self-management and coping strategies that work for them:

> *I run up and down the beach. I use that as a way of getting rid of the frustration and the anger and just a temper, I just run and run and run until I can't run anymore, just, you know, rather than going home and screaming and shouting at her [partner], because I just feel rough as a road, I just feel like just punishing myself. I know I shouldn't because I know I'm going to pay for it in the long run, but at the moment it's just my release, you know. I don't hurt anybody else, I just stick my headphones on and I can just run, run, and run. I get home and I'm like exhausted, but it's ... yeah, I think you need a release from it. (Steve, 44yrs, rheumatoid arthritis, White British)* (Flurey et al., 2016b)

7.4 Just Get on with It

The idea that you've got to *"just get on with it"* (Robert, 60yrs, rheumatoid arthritis, White British) was common throughout both my own studies and the literature in response to managing living with a long-term condition. Many men were reluctant to dwell on the difficulties and instead focused on the importance of carrying on regardless. It was rare to hear men explicitly express the expectation to 'man up' but this sentiment was echoed throughout narratives with emphasis placed on carrying on despite physical or emotional barriers. The man in the following quote seems to take pride in his ability to carry on, and uses language that minimises the emotional impact of a cancer diagnosis:

> *I clicked into a zone. ... From the day I was diagnosed, you know? I had a little bit of a bloke meltdown. ... But the next day I was up and I was like 'OK, what do I have to do today?' (AM18, born 1950s, cancer, Aboriginal Australian)* (Newman et al., 2017)

Men seemed to be motivated to keep going for a variety of reasons. Some had more intrinsic motivation such as the desire to be independent, self-sufficient, competent, and retain as much control over their lives as possible. Some men with cancer discussed the importance for them to keep exercising as it was one of the few behaviours still under their control:

> *Off the top of my head, probably exercise mainly for taking back or holding onto what the cancer took from me. You have to work harder to hold onto what remains. That makes me feel empowered as a man. (P3, prostate cancer, Canada)* (Langelier et al., 2022)

Other men discussed more extrinsic motivation to keep going such as a sense of responsibility to be the breadwinner or maintain their social or family roles (as discussed in Chap. 2). For some men, having a faith helped give their lives meaning and provided them with a reason to keep going. Across the literature many men also discuss trying to limit the burden on their families, which can add pressure to find ways to keep going. George discusses how he deals with this by pacing himself to ensure he can still participate:

George *You've got to pace yourself, you know if you don't. Like you say, holidays, the wife … say like Benidorm, I'll go up on the bus and she'll walk up and I'll walk back, but I can't walk up and walk back, so it's all little things like that that you know you've got to do otherwise you don't enjoy your holiday, do you?*

Tom *No, that's right.*

George *I think because you've had it for a few years now, you've adapted to what you know you've got to do, whether you like it or not, you just know that if you go against or go the opposite way you just … you're ruining their holiday as well.*
(Focus group with men with systemic sclerosis, UK)

My previous work in rheumatoid arthritis with predominantly female participants found that patients find ways to work around their condition through using tools and devices or adapting their environment to make their lives easier (Flurey et al., 2014b). Men also do this but in addition to using tools they had bought or were given in occupational therapy, many also seemed to craft their own devices to make their lives easier. I will discuss how this could feed into developing support for men in Chap. 9:

> *I couldn't pull the clutch lever in on the motorbike, so I made one that was an inch longer. You know, you've got to find ways. (David, 58yrs, rheumatoid arthritis, White British)*

Men often said that they find it difficult to ask for help, and some would resist as much as possible. However, others had begun to accept that asking for help could enable them to keep going and do the things they wanted to. There may be strength to be found in overcoming the obstacle of requesting help:

> *I try to find a way to keep moving to keep doing it and whatever I can, and if I get to the point to ask for help, okay, I ask for help. I have to keep moving and keep doing the things that I have to do, I cannot sit down and just get depressed and, you know, not do anything. That's, at least, that's not the way I am, right? (Jorge, 49yrs, systemic sclerosis, Latino)*

7.5 Becoming an Expert

Most men were keen to have a better understanding of their condition and how to manage it. In a systematic literature review looking at support needs for men with long-term conditions, men have been described as *"hungry for information"* (Galdas et al., 2014). In the focus group setting men tended to be interested in sharing experiences and learning from each other and were often keen to share their expertise. Men sought out various sources to help them develop their knowledge. Some men used message boards and social media such as Facebook groups to learn from and connect with other patients. However, others highlighted the accuracy of this information couldn't be trusted and discussed experiences of reading things that scared or upset them. Research focusing on social media interactions in relation to men's health is limited. However, a recent study found that whilst men's health is a popular topic on Instagram and TikTok, there was a low level of accuracy in health information (Dubin et al., 2022). Social media platforms such as X (formerly Twitter), Threads, and Reddit also provide spaces for men to discuss their experiences or to 'follow' experts allowing them to keep up with the most up-to-date information. However, some men favoured more traditionally reputable sources of information such as journal articles, or material provided by disease-specific patient charities.

Men also sought information from their specialist consultant or wider multidisciplinary team and often respected their level of knowledge and experience. Due to the nature of long-term conditions being managed over time, patients often build a relationship with their clinical team. Many men seemed to value their clinicians getting to know them well enough to pitch information at a level they would understand it. In this way some men praised their clinicians for simplifying complex information into lay language, whilst others valued being treated as intellectual equals and mentioned being given journal articles to read. Some men explained their clinicians had involved them as exemplar patients in specialist training, and there seemed to be an element of pride in contributing to clinician education.

However, not all men found they were able to gain the information they needed from their clinical team. The following exchange is in response to being asked where they get their information about their condition; note the 'doctor' being referred to is their general practitioner (GP):

Alfie *Definitely not the doctor.*
Tim *No, the doctor doesn't really, I've got a new doctor and she's very nice and she does understand it, but she doesn't know much about it as such and I think that's probably what you find everywhere, you know,*
Alfie *The doctors are good, they see me straight away but, you know, 'when are you going back to the [specialist hospital] next, can you wait till then', 'oh'.*
(Focus group with men with systemic sclerosis, UK)

Systemic sclerosis is a rare condition with multiple complex symptoms that differ across patients. It was therefore a common (and perhaps unsurprising) experience for men with systemic sclerosis that their GP would refer them to their rheumatology team for complex questions. Thus, many men had the feeling they had more expertise in their condition than their GP. However, Alfie goes on to say that he still doesn't find he gets the answers he needs from his rheumatology team. He explains that he doesn't remember to ask everything he needs to in the consultation and so will supplement his knowledge through Facebook groups. Alfie is recently widowed and therefore attends his consultations on his own. In Chap. 9 I'll discuss the role family play in supporting men, which can include supporting them in gathering information in consultations, and consider how to better support unpartnered men like Alfie:

Alfie *You have to ask them the right question, but sometimes you don't always remember.*
Tim *Yes, yeah.*
Alfie *When you left you think, 'oh I didn't ask that'. You go online, Facebook straight away, someone always comes in and you get three or four, they're all the same answers and you think, 'ah, that's what I need to do'.*
(Focus group with men with systemic sclerosis, UK)

In terms of the type of information sought, Wenger and Oliffe (2013) found that men with cancer focused on four key areas: understanding their disease (e.g., origin, functioning, and medical terminology), making wise decisions (e.g., regarding treatment options), resolving the disease's impacts (e.g., physical and emotional self-management and coping skills), and re-envisioning their future (e.g., seeking information about the long-term course, survival odds). Although identified in men with cancer, these four areas of information need are familiar throughout my own research and the rest of the long-term conditions literature and can be seen throughout the dialogue in the current chapter, and throughout this book.

7.6 Avoidance and Apathy

In contrast to actively seeking out information to help them understand or manage their condition, some men will choose avoidance or apathy. It is worth highlighting that it is too simplistic to place men into two separate groups of those who use active or passive management of their condition. Depending on the stage they are at in their diagnosis, or how they are feeling on a particular day, men can at different times adopt both of these types of coping interchangeably.

Some men reported an element of apathy or fatalism towards their condition. These men may adhere to their medication regime but beyond that didn't make any changes to their lifestyles and were resigned to feeling unable to help themselves. This was particularly apparent in the diabetes literature, which may reflect societal attitudes and health beliefs. Type 2 diabetes may not be perceived as serious or life threatening in the same way as, for example, cancer:

> *Well I just … I didn't know too much about diabetes, but I didn't feel bad or nothing. Just taking my medication. I ain't changed nothing from what I've been doing. I'm doing everything I [have] been doing. (type 2 diabetes, African American)* (Walker et al., 2022)

Fatalism was also sometimes linked to religious or spiritual beliefs in those men who believed in leaving this to fate or God's will. A meta-analysis of qualitative literature in prostate cancer suggests these beliefs were more commonly explicitly stated by Latin Americans. For some men, this belief freed them up to focus on living rather than thinking about dying:

I know it's not gonna spread any faster than God will let it spread. (Latin American, Prostate cancer) (Rivas et al., 2016)

Some men discussed engaging in avoidant behaviours and sought ways to distract themselves from thinking about their condition. This helped in not dwelling on things that are worrying them but may also prevent them from confronting or addressing their emotions. In moderation or for the short term, avoidance can be a protective coping strategy, but prolonged reliance on this can be linked to distress and depression. The following quote from a man with prostate cancer explains how he uses exercise. Whilst exercise can be a helpful self-management strategy to maintain a healthy body, this man describes using exercise as a way of suppressing or avoiding his emotions. If used as the only coping strategy for emotions this could have the potential to lead to the 'big build' of negative emotions described in Chap. 3:

> *Exercise is a great way to just get out of the house and walk away from things. If I'm going to cry, which is an uncomfortable and uncharacteristic thing to do … either sitting in another room or going out is the best. (P10, prostate cancer, Canada)* (Langelier et al., 2022)

Avoidance shouldn't be confused with escapism. Some men discussed choosing to take space to collect their thoughts and acknowledge their emotions. In the next section I will cover how men will open up to others in the right circumstances. Men often feel responsible for those close to them and therefore it may be important to have space to collect their thoughts before talking to others as this comes with the added complexity of the other person's potential emotional response. Kevin talks about how fishing provides him with a cover for precious time to reflect:

> *I'd go and sit in the freezing cold pretending to fish … gave me time to think about everything an' I needed that sometimes just to sit and think about where I was what was comin' what the possibilities were, rather than let things build up so fishing was an escape. (Kevin, breast cancer, UK)* (Quincey et al., 2021)

7.7 Selective Disclosure

Men talking about the emotional impact of living with a long-term condition has been discussed in Chap. 3. This section will focus on men talking about their condition more broadly, as a form of coping or self-management.

When asked whether they disclose their condition to other people or talk about the impact on their lives, many men often at first say they don't talk about it at all. However, on further discussion it seems that men may simply be selective in who they trust to talk to. Some men choose not to tell people as they don't think other people will understand what they're going through, some felt uncomfortable receiving sympathy from others or wanted to avoid being looked at with pity, some didn't want to be seen to be complaining or worried that they would be seen as boring by talking about their troubles. Black African and Black Caribbean men explained that they are brought up not to share negative experiences, which may be important for not showing weakness to others and maintaining masculine status:

> *You don't confess the negative, so you're not taught to say: oh, I'm having a headache. Yeah? Say: Oh, it is well with me, rather than say: oh I have a splitting migraine, can you do something about that? … They have to be positive always, … without actually analysing what is happening and doing what is right. (Participant 5, prostate cancer, Black African)* (Wagland et al., 2019)

There were mixed responses on whether men would disclose their long-term condition to an employer with some feeling they had no choice due to needing time off for appointments, or for insurance purposes, and others choosing to conceal their condition due to embarrassment or worries about discrimination or missing out on opportunities (as discussed in Chap. 2). Whilst some men felt able to disclose their condition to their male friends or co-workers, others concealed it as they didn't want to be the focus of cruel and hurtful comments in the guise of 'male banter'. James explains below that his friends were initially supportive and showed concern, but soon reverted to expecting him to keep up with them when the immediate serious threat to health was no longer so apparent:

> *When I first went in hospital with it and all the rest of it, all my mates wanted to know what was going on and all about it, and they would sit … well, they did, they sat sort of intently listening to all the … what happened here and what*

> *happened there, but now, erm, if I mention … I go [clay] shooting every Saturday afternoon right, clay shooting and if I complain just for a minute like, to say hold on, I'm … you know, I've got arthritis … they'll say 'stop bloody moaning'. That's all you get. You know, they've sort of … we've gone past it where they'll listen. (James, 72yrs, rheumatoid arthritis, White British)* (Flurey et al., 2016b)

As discussed in Chap. 3, the emotional impact can be harder for men to talk about than the physical. Men generally said they would talk to their clinical team but interestingly when I pushed them on this, they expressed that they would focus on the physical symptoms even when the emotional side is what was bothering them. It is worth reiterating the point I made in Chap. 3 that it is important for clinicians to directly ask men about the emotional impact, especially if they present with physical symptoms when their condition would medically be considered well-controlled.

Throughout this book I have demonstrated that men can and do talk when given the opportunity and the right conditions, but they may be selective about how much they share and with whom. Men most often said they would talk to their wives or partners, and for unpartnered men they often valued adult daughters or female friends for emotional support. Whilst some men would talk to their male friends, and most would at least let close friends know they had a long-term condition (*"You don't have to go into much detail, just, sorry I can't be like I used to be"*, Henry, 78yrs, systemic sclerosis, White British) they often seemed to be negotiating social rules of how much it would be acceptable to share:

> *There's always a limit to what you talk about. There's never a full-blown conversation about feelings and emotions but there always is in some sort of form … you can speak openly more to some than others. (Henry, 25yrs, anxiety, Welsh)* (Gough et al., 2021)

While many men will most readily talk about their experiences with close (often female) relatives, they also expressed masking the full impact of their condition as they seemed to feel responsible for not burdening them. Some based this on previous experiences and wanted to avoid their partners becoming distressed over being unable to help them or cause them any additional worries. Others perceived they had a responsibility to protect those close to them and chose to conceal things that had the potential to upset them:

In terms of talking to the wife, I just, I can't do it anymore, I can't burden her anymore, 'cause she's like a worry person, so if you give her worry it doesn't go. It's just constantly, she's constantly thinking, [...], and like, a lot of times reflux hits me at night time and I, I'm like, [wife] says, 'are you okay?' I say, 'yeah, I'm just going down to get some milk', I run downside and balling out my eyes, and feel like a dragon, the acid is just coming right up to my throat and I go back up the stairs and she goes, 'are you okay?', 'yeah, yeah, I'm alright, I just had a bit of milk, I'm alright'. I can't tell her how I feel, I just can't. (Emil, 37yrs, systemic sclerosis, Black British)

I didn't tell my mum [about his diagnosis] because she would get upset and she lives in another country right, so why bother to tell her if she's like miles away and she's going to get, er, so whatever. (Jorge, 49yrs, systemic sclerosis, Latino)

If men find themselves masking the full impact of their condition from the key supportive people in their lives, this really highlights the importance of providing a way men can feel supported beyond their existing social support structures. For many of the men in my focus group studies, this was the first opportunity they had to speak to other men with the same condition, and even those who expressed they don't usually speak to anyone seemed to value this opportunity to open up about their experiences, and to learn from and support others. However, all the participants are of course those who have chosen to take part in a focus group study and may therefore be more comfortable speaking to a group of other men than those who may not have chosen to take part:

I'm kind of the same way I don't really talk about it to anybody and, you know, obviously your close relatives see, so they know, but in terms of just, er, you know there are not many people that experience the same thing so it's hard to find that connection with somebody. (Bill, 66yrs, systemic sclerosis, White American)

7.8 Positive Focus

Some men talked about their ability to look on the bright side of things, and maintaining a positive outlook seemed to help them cope (*"I've got a cheerful disposition so it takes a lot to put me down"*, Charles, rheumatoid arthritis). This may not work for all men, as pressure to maintain positivity in the face of difficulty can create its own burden. As a way of helping to see the positives in their situation many men made downward comparisons either to other patients or to people in other less fortunate situations (e.g., some mentioned children with cancer). Social comparisons can be a particularly helpful coping strategy when a person is unable to change their situation (Wills, 1981, 1987).

Some men tried to find a positive outlet to focus their energies, which may also serve as a distraction to focusing on their worries about the condition. This included advocacy, activism, charity work, or contributing to support services. Men with breast cancer explained they were motivated by feeling duty-bound to raise awareness, wanting to feel their voice was heard and improve care practices (Quincey et al., 2021), or a sense of personal satisfaction from helping others (Potter et al., 2023).

7.9 Acceptance: Redefining Not Rejecting Masculinity

Some previous studies have suggested that men need to reject or depart from traditional masculinity to cope with and accept living with a long-term condition. However, for many men this seemed to be more of a redefining, renegotiating, or reconstructing of masculinity rather than an all-out rejection. Some men may resist culturally dominant definitions of masculinity, but this seems to be part of a broader attitude towards masculine norms based on their individual values rather than in response to learning to live with a long-term condition (Emslie et al., 2006).

Men who have had some areas of masculinity compromised seem to highlight areas of their lives where they are still able to exert traditional masculine values; for example, George explains that whilst he has lost his libido he would still 'hold his own' as a man if he was challenged:

> *I wouldn't say it still affects my maleness. If somebody did me wrong I would still go for them. … I wouldn't call on my wife to go and fight my battles. (George, coronary heart disease, Scotland)* (O'Brien et al., 2007)

Men's discourses suggested that strength was redefined from physical abilities to the strength to withstand the pain from their condition or undergo invasive treatment. For men with prostate cancer, strength was also found in survival (Alexis & Worsley, 2018). Chris compares the level of pain he has now become used to on a daily basis to how he perceives others would cope with this:

I would say most days you wake up, and anybody who hadn't had this would, erm get up and think, 'oh I better go and see a doctor, er, see my GP', but I just take the pills and carry on really as best you can, and every day is different. (Chris, 55yrs, systemic sclerosis, White British)

As discussed in Chap. 2, masculine values of responsibility were channelled into taking care of their own health and bravado was sometimes used to assert this. Having financial means to pay people to do things for them (e.g., tradesmen) was preferred to accepting favours and helped men to reconcile having to ask other men to do things they used to be able to do for themselves.

7.10 Summary

Societal narratives often accuse men of being poor at looking after their health, but this is an unfair characterisation, particularly in men with long-term conditions. The direct threat to men's health of a diagnosis of a long-term condition for many men can refocus their attention on taking care of not only their symptom management but additionally their overall wellbeing. Men tend to find ways to work around any limitations (often in creative ways) to enable them to carry on with their lives as much as possible. Men are often keen to develop expertise in their condition to help them understand and manage it and have a variety of preferences for how they access this information. At times, men may use avoidance and apathy as coping strategies, which may need attention to ensure this doesn't lead to distress. Men will talk about their condition with trusted others, but clinicians should be aware that men may still mask the full impact from those closest to them making it important to provide support systems beyond men's own social networks. Finally, men do not necessarily need to depart from masculinity to reach acceptance of their condition, and may find value in identifying areas where they can still demonstrate masculinity.

References

Abbott, D., Jepson, M., & Hastie, J. (2016). Men living with long-term conditions: Exploring gender and improving social care. *Health & Social Care in the Community, 24*(4), 420–427. https://doi.org/10.1111/hsc.12222

Alexis, O., & Worsley, A. J. (2018). A meta-synthesis of qualitative studies exploring men's sense of masculinity post-prostate cancer treatment. *Cancer Nursing, 41*(4), 298–310. https://doi.org/10.1097/NCC.0000000000000509

Dubin, J. M., Aguiar, J. A., Lin, J. S., Greenberg, D. R., Keeter, M. K., Fantus, R. J., Pham, M. N., Hudnall, M. T., Bennett, N. E., Brannigan, R. E., & Halpern, J. A. (2022). The broad reach and inaccuracy of men's health information on social media: Analysis of TikTok and Instagram. *International Journal of Impotence Research*, 1–5. https://doi.org/10.1038/s41443-022-00645-6

Emslie, C., Ridge, D., Ziebland, S., & Hunt, K. (2006). Men's accounts of depression: Reconstructing or resisting hegemonic masculinity? *Social Science & Medicine, 62*(9), 2246–2257.

Flurey, C., Pauling, J. D., Saketkoo, L. A., Denton, C. P., Galdas, P., Khanna, D., Williams, A., & Hughes, M. (2022). 'I turned in my man card': A qualitative study of the experiences, coping styles and support needs of men with systemic sclerosis. *Rheumatology, 62*(6), 2160–2167. https://doi.org/10.1093/RHEUMATOLOGY/KEAC585

Galdas, P., Darwin, Z., Kidd, L., Blickem, C., McPherson, K., Hunt, K., Bower, P., Gilbody, S., & Richardson, G. (2014). The accessibility and acceptability of self-management support interventions for men with long term conditions: A systematic review and meta-synthesis of qualitative studies. *BMC Public Health, 14*(1), 1230.

Gough, B., Robertson, S., & Luck, H. (2021). Engendered expressions of anxiety: Men's emotional communications with women and other men. *Frontiers in Sociology, 6*. https://doi.org/10.3389/FSOC.2021.697356

Ireland, D. (2019, August 11). *"Don't confuse your medical degree with my life"—Patient.* LinkedIn. https://www.linkedin.com/pulse/dont-confuse-your-medical-degree-my-life-patient-dawn-m-ireland/

Klafke, N., Eliott, J., Olver, I., & Wittert, G. (2014). Australian men with cancer practice complementary therapies (CTs) as a coping strategy. *Psycho-Oncology, 23*(11), 1236–1242. https://doi.org/10.1002/pon.3550

Langelier, D. M., Jackson, C., Bridel, W., Grant, C., & Culos-Reed, S. N. (2022). Coping strategies in active and inactive men with prostate cancer: A qualitative study. *Journal of Cancer Survivorship, 16*(2), 421–431. https://doi.org/10.1007/S11764-021-01037-3

Lim, S. S., Vos, T., Flaxman, A. D., Danaei, G., Shibuya, K., Adair-Rohani, H., AlMazroa, M. A., Amann, M., Anderson, H. R., & Andrews, K. G. (2012). A comparative risk assessment of burden of disease and injury attributable to 67 risk factors and risk factor clusters in 21 regions, 1990–2010: A systematic analysis for the Global Burden of Disease Study 2010. *The Lancet, 380*(9859), 2224–2260.

Newman, C. E., Gray, R., Brener, L., Jackson, L. C., Dillon, A., Saunders, V., Johnson, P., & Treloar, C. (2017). "I had a little bit of a bloke meltdown…But the next day, i was up": Understanding cancer experiences among aboriginal men. *Cancer Nursing, 40*(3), E1–E8. https://doi.org/10.1097/NCC.0000000000000399

O'Brien, R., Hart, G. J., & Hunt, K. (2007). "Standing out from the herd": Men renegotiating masculinity in relation to their experience of illness. *International Journal of Men's Health, 6*(3), 178–200.

Oliffe, J. L., Rasmussen, B., Bottorff, J. L., Kelly, M. T., Galdas, P. M., Phinney, A., & Ogrodniczuk, J. S. (2013). Masculinities, work, and retirement among older men who experience depression. *Qualitative Health Research, 23*(12), 1626–1637. https://doi.org/10.1177/1049732313509408

Potter, A. M., Bentz, B., Crue, L., Leiby, S., Bashi, S., Maguire, K., Meyers, J., & Mieczkowski, K. (2023). Men's lived experiences of breast cancer and changes in occupation. *Occupational Therapy International.* https://doi.org/10.1155/2023/9641922

Quincey, K., Williamson, I., & Wildbur, D. (2021). Men with breast cancer and their encounters with masculinity: An interpretative phenomenological analysis using photography. *Psychology of Men and Masculinity, 22*(4), 690–703. https://doi.org/10.1037/MEN0000344

Rivas, C., Matheson, L., Nayoan, J., Glaser, A., Gavin, A., Wright, P., Wagland, R., & Watson, E. (2016). Ethnicity and the prostate cancer experience: A qualitative metasynthesis. In *Psycho-Oncology* (Vol. 25, Issue 10, pp. 1147–1156). https://doi.org/10.1002/pon.4222

Robertson, S., Sheikh, K., & Moore, A. (2010). Embodied masculinities in the context of cardiac rehabilitation. *Sociology of Health & Illness, 32*(5), 695–710. https://doi.org/10.1111/j.1467-9566.2010.01249.x

Wagland, R., Nayoan, J., Matheson, L., Rivas, C., Brett, J., Collaco, N., Alexis, O., Gavin, A., Glaser, A. W., & Watson, E. (2019). Adjustment strategies amongst black African and black Caribbean men following treatment for prostate cancer: Findings from the Life After Prostate Cancer Diagnosis. *European Journal of Cancer Care, 29*(1). https://doi.org/10.1111/ecc.13183

Walker, A. Q., Blake, C. E., Moore, J. B., Wilcox, S., DuBois, K., Watkins, W., & K. (2022). Experiences of midlife and older African American men living with type 2 diabetes. *Ethnicity & Health, 27*(6), 1256–1270. https://doi.org/10.1080/13557858.2021.1910206

Wenger, L., & Oliffe, J. (2013). Men managing cancer: A gender analysis. *Sociology of Health & Illness, 36*(1), 108–122. https://doi.org/10.1111/1467-9566.12045

Wills, T. A. (1981). Downward comparison principles in social psychology. *Psychological Bulletin, 90*(2), 245–271.

Wills, T. A. (1987). Downward comparison as a coping mechanism. In C. R. Snyder & C. Ford (Eds.), *Coping with negative life events: Clinical and social-psychological perspectives*. Plenum Press.

CHAPTER 8

Help-Seeking

"*Before I was diagnosed I didn't even know what my doctor looked like*".

Whenever I tell people that my work focuses on men's health, the most common response I receive is a knowing "ah yes, because men don't go to the doctor". This is such a prevailing narrative in society that men themselves often subscribe to it, and resisting seeking medical help can itself be used as a marker of masculinity. Courtenay (2000) suggests men and boys may reject healthy beliefs and behaviours as a way of demonstrating masculinity. Thus, by dismissing their health needs and emphasising a lack of engagement with healthcare they are constructing gender to situate themselves in a masculine arena.

In my own focus groups and throughout the literature, men's narratives indicated an acknowledgement of this expectation for men not to seek medical help, suggesting subscribing to masculine norms as the reason for this:

> *Machoism isn't it really …? It's … tough guys don't need help. (prostate cancer, UK)* (Medina-Perucha et al., 2017)

It seemed to be important to men to highlight that although they may now be under regular clinical care due to a long-term condition, this was not usual for them prior to their diagnosis. This narrative implies their health behaviours are the same as other men and this is an exceptional

C. Flurey, *Talking Men's Health*,
https://doi.org/10.1007/978-3-031-62593-0_8

circumstance—taking responsibility for their health would be the natural response for any man facing a serious health condition. This reinforcement of their previous alignment with traditionally masculine ways of approaching health may help with reconciling these new health behaviours within a masculine identity:

Robert *Before I was diagnosed, I didn't even know what my doctor looked like.*

James *You just got to get on with it. … Well, I was the same.*

Robert *I never went to the doctor.*

James *I hadn't been to my doctor … in fact, I had to change my doctor because I was still registered with an old surgery down in [redacted], and he said, where have you been, he said, we have no record of you doing anything for the last 15 years.*

Robert *That's right, yes, you don't see them, men don't go to the doctor, do they?*

(Focus group with men with systemic sclerosis, UK).

8.1 Are Men as Bad at Seeking Help as We Think?

It is widely acknowledged that men don't visit their general practitioner (GP) as often as women in early adulthood (White & Banks, 2009). This may be unsurprising when we consider there are various reproductive reasons that may result in higher numbers of GP visits for women, but the picture is slightly more complex than this.

A study conducted in Spain used medical records from 79,809 adult patients who attended primary healthcare services at least once in 2008. They found the gross number of visits to primary care was higher in women. However, when adjusting for age and morbidity burden, there was no difference in primary care visits between women and men (Carretero et al., 2014). Thus, whilst women may have a higher total number of primary care visits, this would suggest they are related to clinical need rather than men's reluctance to seek help. Looking at everyday pain, a literature review of help-seeking behaviours for back pain and headaches found no consistent evidence of greater consultation among women for back pain than for men. There was some evidence that women consult more for headaches than men, but this wasn't consistent across the literature (Hunt et al., 2011).

By contrast, a large-scale study in Denmark based on 35.8 million GP contacts and 1.2 million hospitalisations in 2005 found men were less likely to contact their GP but more likely to be hospitalised and had higher mortality rates (Juel & Christensen, 2008). This would align with the theory that men delay help-seeking for severe symptoms, meaning they are more likely to have worse outcomes (hospitalisation or death). However, a cross-sectional study assessed medical records of patients in the UK who had been diagnosed with colorectal cancer (n = 12,189), lung cancer (n = 11,081), or malignant melanoma (n = 4352) and found no significant gender differences in the percentage of patients who consulted their GP, and the number of GP contacts made in the 24 months prior to diagnosis (Wang et al., 2014). It is also worth noting that analysis of data from a US health report suggests women are more likely to receive preventative healthcare services from primary care than age-matched male controls over age 15 years (White, 2007). This provides compelling evidence to suggest the reasons for higher hospitalisation and mortality rates in men may be far more complex than men delaying help-seeking for serious issues longer than women.

Thus, it seems that overall men may not be so much worse at seeking medical help than women. The assumption that women will more readily seek medical help than men may be perpetuating a harmful stereotype that health concerns are women's domain, and 'real men' are unconcerned with their health. Additionally, these assumptions may contribute to unconscious bias in healthcare providers' assessments of symptoms, diagnosis, and clinical management for women if they are assumed to consult at a lower level of symptom severity (Hunt et al., 2011). However, this doesn't mean we can jump to the conclusion that men are good at seeking help and we don't need to worry about them. Across a range of health conditions including HIV and AIDS, cancer, chest pain, and mental health issues, men are reported to delay help-seeking from healthcare services (White & Banks, 2009). Rather than men being the problematic gender, it is likely men and women have different barriers to seeking help. It is important to understand the reasons that men delay help-seeking as they may need different health promotion strategies to women to encourage them to seek help sooner.

8.2 Barriers to Help-Seeking for Men with Long-Term Conditions

A key reason (common to both men and women) for delaying help-seeking is not recognising the symptoms they are experiencing as a sign of something serious, or symptoms not causing sufficient discomfort or disruption to daily life to warrant attention. This may be particularly likely to delay men's help-seeking in conditions that affect more women than men or are considered 'women's conditions' as men may be less familiar with the early warning signs. For example, in breast cancer this was the predominant reason men delayed help-seeking, whilst otherwise reporting fairly prompt medical help-seeking once recognising symptoms as a cause for concern (Quincey et al., 2016). Interviews with men with lung cancer indicate that they may assess the risk of symptoms as less serious than clinicians, which can contribute to refusal or delays in accepting treatment:

> *I just seen a spot on the X-ray. A little bitty spot and I'm a big man. It'd take a lot to pull me down. (lung cancer, USA)* (Sharf et al., 2005)

This idea that men will delay help-seeking while they try and make sense of their symptoms has also been found in men experiencing chest pain (White & Johnson, 2000). Men in this study waited to seek help for their symptoms beyond the point that would be expected by the clinical team. The authors suggest that men are not prepared to deal with a body changing from healthy to ill. To reach the point of seeking help men may have to reconcile deep-seated feelings of invincibility with a new and unexpected threat to their health. This process may be new and uncomfortable for men experiencing symptoms of an acute condition, or prior to diagnosis of a long-term condition. However, having been through this process during diagnosis, coupled with previous positive experiences of help-seeking, some men with long-term conditions do report readily seeking help for exacerbation of ongoing symptoms:

> *If I get a flare up then I usually contact the rheumatoid clinic [...] and they either, erm ... give me an injection of steroids or put me on steroids which within a couple of days it's all back to normal again. (Mark, 49yrs, rheumatoid arthritis, White British)*

I should point out that my own work in rheumatoid arthritis (with both men and women) found patients often saw seeking help as a last resort and would exhaust all self-management strategies before contacting their medical team for help (Flurey et al., 2014a, 2014b). Thus, it is possible that when participants talk about seeking help quickly this may be in relation to the amount of time since assessing symptoms as unmanageable, rather than shortly after experiencing the first symptoms. Thus, it may still be longer than would be expected or advised by healthcare professionals.

The desire or expectation to conform to hegemonic masculine standards also seems to play an integral role in men's help-seeking behaviours. Men sampled across a variety of life experiences report a reluctance to seek help (or to be seen to be seeking help) due to concerns that this would make them seem 'less of a man'. This was particularly seen in younger 'healthy' participants where they may still be negotiating their developing masculine identities and looking to male peers for what is acceptable. For many men being seen to be 'strong and silent' or able to endure pain was seen as an important marker of masculinity (O'Brien et al., 2005). However, as I've previously discussed in this book, men who experience illness begin to redefine masculinity to include taking responsibility for their health. This is often framed in terms of reducing the burden on those closest to them, emphasising the protector role of masculinity.

Men often describe being cautious of seeking help for minor symptoms that other men may more readily endure as this may call their masculinity into question (O'Brien et al., 2005). The quote below from Damaa, who positions himself as a "strong man", illustrates this delay in help-seeking until he was in so much pain he had to be hospitalised, at which point his prostate cancer symptoms were sufficiently advanced to be beyond treatment:

> *I've always been a strong man. I don't fall sick often. So, I didn't pay attention to my symptoms until I experienced severe pains and had to be taken to the hospital by my mother. Hmmm … the results broke my heart; the doctors said if I'd reported early, they could have done surgery to remove it, but it was too late now. (Damaa, prostate cancer, Ghanaian)* (Salifu et al., 2023)

Masculine norms in some cultures may emphasise this expectation for men to resist seeking help until it can no longer be avoided. Interviews with Aboriginal Australian men described a culture of staying 'strong and silent' in the face of illness, and managing their own health without medical assistance for as long as possible (Newman et al., 2017):

> *I don't know if it's because I [feel] ashamed to go to the doctors, or [if we] think we're doctors and diagnose ourselves. ... [But] we'd have to be half dead in bed, do you know what I mean? (born 1970s, cancer, Aboriginal Australian)* (Newman et al., 2017)

In addition to concerns about how they would be viewed by their social groups or communities, some men also worried about how they would be perceived by the clinical team if they sought help unnecessarily. Men with fibromyalgia-type pain reported being *"afraid of being looked upon as a whiner"* and therefore putting up with a large amount of pain before seeking help. Some men continued working to the point they collapsed and were hospitalised (Paulson et al., 2002). This reinforces the importance of clinicians validating men's experiences, with dismissal of pain or symptoms having the potential to cause men to further delay help-seeking in the future.

Men with breast cancer often experienced this delay in diagnosis due to the rarity of the condition in men, with men often left feeling frustrated and that their symptoms weren't taken seriously (Quincey et al., 2016). An Aboriginal Australian man with bowel cancer describes how although he did seek help at first, initial dismissal of his symptoms by his GP caused him to delay help-seeking until his symptoms were much more serious:

> *I told [my GP] about different symptoms I had ... and he put it down to stress and irritable bowel syndrome ... when I come to here, I had really bad stomach pains [but] I sort of kept putting it off. ... The pain got really worse and [my new GP] sent me straight to see the gastroenterologist. ... He thought I was too young, so he said he wasn't expecting to find anything too nasty, but as soon as I come out after the [colonoscopy], he told me, 'Yeah, there's a large cancer there that's come through the bowel wall, so we need to get you into surgery straight away!' ... So that's why I am really cranky about that [initial] doctor. (born 1960s, bowel cancer, Aboriginal Australian)* (Newman et al., 2017)

Beyond men's concerns about other people's perceptions of them for seeking help, some men also resisted medical consultations due to avoiding receiving a diagnosis. For some this was due to the fear of having an unwelcome diagnosis confirmed. Some men worried about the stigma associated with a diagnosis, or the impact on their masculinity:

> *I didn't want a diagnosis at first you see. I simply wanted to carry on playing football with the lads and going to the pub. I couldn't say no because that would be embarrassing and they (his friends) would just take the mick and tell me to 'man up'. (Paul, 42yrs, chronic fatigue syndrome, White British)* (Snell et al., 2023)

Other barriers to help-seeking included embarrassment, anxiety, distress, or fear of using healthcare services (Yousaf et al., 2013). For some men, gatekeepers (such as receptionists) presented additional barriers to negotiating these feelings towards seeking help. For some men, these reasons contributed to a resistance to potential treatment options, which could be due to fear or a refusal to accept the impact of this on their identity and quality of life:

> *The receptionist asks you what you want to see the doctor about. Well, I'm not going to tell her I can't get an erection, am I? I don't think they should do that. It's embarrassing enough, but to tell a receptionist why you want to go and see a doctor for. I would never tell her. (prostate cancer, UK)* (Medina-Perucha et al., 2017)

> *As for that operation [removal of the testes], I've ruled it out. It was out of the options for me from day one. Eii [exclamation] taking my testes out will mean I'm no longer a man. The balls make us men, you know. (Maegyida, Ghanaian, prostate cancer)* (Salifu et al., 2023)

Whilst in the UK we are lucky to still have the NHS, it is worth mentioning that in many countries a prominent barrier to seeking medical help was the cost:

> *You know sometimes we put off going to the doctor because we don't have that green stuff to go pay them. (type 2 diabetes, African American)* (Walker et al., 2022)

8.3 Distrust of Medical Professionals in Marginalised Groups

Men are not an homogeneous group, and whilst many barriers to help-seeking may have commonalities across men, experiences of men from marginalised groups cannot be ignored as contributing factors to delayed help-seeking within these communities.

In one study, African American men describe their distrust with medication and medical professionals as primarily based on the awareness of historic unethical experiments and lack of concern for the rights of Black people in the name of 'science'. One participant mentions the Tuskegee syphilis experiments as an example of why people from Black communities have a distrust of white medical professionals and scientists. The Tuskegee syphilis study (1932–1972) looked at the natural course of untreated syphilis in African American men. Participants were not told they had syphilis or that the disease could be transmitted through sexual intercourse. Despite penicillin being discovered in the mid-1940s, treatment was withheld from participants to study the disease until their deaths. It is hardly surprising that this cultural memory of the treatment of Black people by the hands of medical professionals leaves a profound mark of mistrust:

> *From the Black experience, there's a distrust. There's a, there's a distrust and, "Why are you gonna give me that? I know what they do with those Tuskegee men". (male mental health advocate, African American)* (Yaklin et al., 2022)

Whilst we would hope that unethical experiments remain a shameful part of medicine's history, racism still persists in healthcare both explicitly and implicitly. This can take the form of inadequate care and a dismissal of symptoms or suffering, a lack of respect, or a lack of power to negotiate in healthcare interactions. Some healthcare staff stereotype minoritised ethnic groups, characterising them as 'irrational, difficult, frustrating, emotional, or dramatic'. Studies looking at implicit racial bias show that healthcare staff may exhibit racial bias in favour of majority groups, resulting in minoritised groups receive deprioritised diagnoses and treatment. Minoritised groups can also receive inadequate support for treatment choices such as pain medications. These experiences understandably contribute to a loss of trust in healthcare, higher unmet needs, and subsequent delays to help-seeking (Hamed et al., 2022).

Health inequalities in treatment can also contribute to a more negative experience of care for minoritised groups. For example, men with diabetes expressed concerns of treatments not being geared towards African Americans. They were aware that fewer Black patients take part in clinical trials than white patients and questioned how effective medications would be for them (Walker et al., 2022). The recent national early inflammatory arthritis audit found that although a higher proportion of Black, Asian, and minoritised ethnic patients were referred to rheumatology within three working days of presenting to primary care compared to white patients, a lower proportion reported disease remission by three month follow up. Further, a higher proportion reported symptoms of anxiety or depression compared to white patients (British Society for Rheumatology & Health Quality Improvement Partnership, 2022). This indicates that whilst referrals may be improving, there is still a gap in delivering effective care for Black, Asian, and minoritised ethnic patients once they reach Secondary or Tertiary care.

There is limited research on healthcare experiences of men with long-term conditions from LGBTQIA+ communities. However, distrust in medical professionals was also expressed by gay and transgender men, usually based on prior experiences. Some men had experienced direct discrimination due to their sexuality, which put them off future help-seeking behaviours. This overt discrimination may be more pronounced in some cultures than others. Men who have sex with men in Rwanda described discrimination and humiliation (*"[T]hey told me to go home and repent because I'm a sinner"* (Isano et al., 2023)) or were left untreated due to healthcare professionals' lack of knowledge and skills. One man describes this affecting his help-seeking behaviours to the point he would ask a friend to engage with healthcare services on his behalf and source medication privately:

> *Many healthcare providers mistreat us, and exhibit stigma. I decided to stop going to the health facilities, instead I send a friend to the health center on my behalf when sick or I consult my friends in our MSM [men who have sex with men] community for information about medications I can buy in private pharmacy. (22yrs, Rwanda)* (Isano et al., 2023)

Although such overt discrimination may be less common in Western countries, men from LGBTQIA+ communities often still experience discriminatory behaviours from healthcare professionals that affects their care. This can cause fears and reluctance to disclose their sexual orientation or gender identity to healthcare professionals. Worries about having to face negative attitudes and the impact this will have on their care can cause them to delay help-seeking (Ayhan et al., 2020). Gay men can also experience marginalisation through healthcare professionals' lack of knowledge or training for their specific needs. Men with prostate cancer described wanting to have candid discussions with healthcare professionals about the impact on their lives in the context of their sexuality. However, they often perceived healthcare professionals had little understanding of their experiences or needs. One participant described delaying surgery until he found a surgeon who was willing to listen to his concerns and agree to perform nerve-sparing surgery (Doran et al., 2018). This reinforces the importance of clinicians understanding the specific needs and barriers of marginalised groups, and the need for training to improve healthcare support for these communities.

8.4 Encouraging Men to Seek Help

Across my own research and the literature men frequently discuss their family (often but not limited to spouses and partners) being integral to prompting them to seek medical help. I discussed this in Chap. 3 in relation to depression, using the example of Frank who was prompted by his son to seek help. Families also perform an integral role in prompting men to seek help for physical symptoms:

> *I was working for about six months with it and I was waking up in the morning, some days I couldn't, it was a squeeze to get my boots on and I just carried on working and working and working. My missus ... I came home one day and she just turned around and said, 'You've got to go to the hospital otherwise you're going to end up falling apart otherwise.' It was a bit of a shock, I burst into tears in front of the doctor when he finally told me what it was because I really thought that it was just old age, I thought ... he turned around and said, 'You're not old.' (Steve, 44yrs, rheumatoid arthritis, White British)*

For some men, consulting friends or family members before seeking help for physical symptoms was a way of 'checking' that their symptoms were severe enough to warrant attention. This legitimised their concerns and confirmed they were not over-reacting (O'Brien et al., 2005). Being encouraged to seek help by a friend or family member may also provide men with the ability to save face and 'blame' their 'overly-concerned' friend or family member should their symptoms turn out to be non-serious.

Men with prostate cancer report consulting their spouses or partners in their decision to undergo prostate cancer screening, and in deciding which treatment options to pursue. Key women in men's lives often help by encouraging doctor visits, scheduling medical appointments, and seeking prostate cancer screening (Bergner et al., 2018).

Friends and family members may therefore play a crucial role in encouraging men to seek help and should be harnessed to support men's health promotion. However, it is important to note that there can be cultural barriers to suggesting to men that they seek medical help. Black African and Black Caribbean men reported the importance of 'pitching' the conversation carefully, as discussion about illness can be interpreted as 'wishing evil' upon someone:

> *As a black person, OK, I have three brothers, oh, I need to tell them. You've got to be careful. How you say that to them. Because the way we're risen is different with respect to negative things. So it will be that they say: oh, so are you wishing me evil. OK? ... Rather than: oh, that's true, maybe I should read about this and try to understand. It is most likely to be interpreted that you're wishing them evil. ... So with black communities one has got to understand the audience very well in order to pitch that presentation. (Participant 2, 70yrs, prostate cancer, Black African)* (Wagland et al., 2019)

Whilst friends and family members can play an integral role in men's help-seeking behaviours it is important to remember that not all men are partnered or have close friends. Thus, we need to look beyond this as a strategy to engaging men. Throughout this book I have discussed how men with long-term conditions seem to renegotiate their definitions of masculinity to find strength in taking responsibility for their health and having self-awareness of their bodies. This harnessing of positive masculine traits to reinforce the idea that seeking help demonstrates masculine strength would be a helpful message for men at all life stages:

> *Because I'm disabled and I'm a man, I think you're more of a man if you accept that you need help. That's strength. It's not a weakness. I need to accept care. I think that men use tools and stuff. Carers are like the tools to help you in your life, really. (Duchenne muscular dystrophy, UK)* (Abbott et al., 2016)

Advocates for men's health sometimes use the narrative that men's health is ignored by healthcare professionals, with positive intentions to raise awareness of the need to provide tailored support to men. However, as the below quote demonstrates this can have unintentional negative consequences by reinforcing men's concerns that if they seek help for minor symptoms they will be dismissed. Thus, it may be important to ensure that men's health promotion includes the messaging that they will be taken seriously—and crucially that this is carried into practice. It is important for clinicians to understand that men have often waited and given much thought to whether their symptoms are severe enough before seeking help:

> *There has been so much publicity on how males are not taken seriously when they admit how they are feeling, so this puts me off going. (Sam, 32yrs, chronic fatigue syndrome, White British) (Snell et al.,* 2023*)*

Finally, encouraging men to seek medical help can mean making it as easy as possible for them to engage with health services through placing these in the communities that they routinely reside and frequent (Oliffe et al., 2020). Health promotion (e.g., to encourage screening behaviours) can be particularly effective when placed in community settings that men are familiar with and trust the knowledge and advice of community leaders within that setting:

> *Barber shops would be a good place to promote health education and health promotion about the taboos and also churches. In talking to men in barber shops, you would be surprised at how much they know. They are very aware. (prostate cancer, African/Afro-Caribbean)* (Anderson et al., 2013)

Designing services that encourage men to engage with them will be discussed further in the next chapter.

8.5 Summary

Despite social narratives, men may not be any worse at seeking help for serious symptoms than women. However, men do still delay in consulting healthcare services for a variety of reasons. These include assessing whether their symptoms are sufficiently serious to warrant seeking help, and concerns over being seen by others as weak for seeking help unnecessarily. Other reasons include fear and embarrassment of the healthcare process or resulting outcomes such as diagnosis or surgery. Men may also be put off seeking help by previous negative experiences such as symptoms being dismissed, or direct or indirect discrimination. Men may be encouraged to seek help by being prompted by a friend or family member, the message that men will be taken seriously by healthcare services (and following through on this), and services being embedded in their communities. Designing services tailored to men will be discussed in the following chapter.

References

Abbott, D., Jepson, M., & Hastie, J. (2016). Men living with long-term conditions: Exploring gender and improving social care. *Health & Social Care in the Community, 24*(4), 420–427. https://doi.org/10.1111/hsc.12222

Anderson, B., Marshall-Lucette, S., & Webb, P. (2013). African and Afro-Caribbean men's experiences of prostate cancer. *British Journal of Nursing, 22*(22), 1296–1307. https://doi.org/10.12968/BJON.2013.22.22.1296

Ayhan, C. H. B., Bilgin, H., Uluman, O. T., Sukut, O., Yilmaz, S., & Buzlu, S. (2020). A systematic review of the discrimination against sexual and gender minority in health care settings. *International Journal of Health Services, 50*(1), 44–61. https://doi.org/10.1177/0020731419885093

Bergner, E. M., Cornish, E. K., Horne, K., & Griffith, D. M. (2018). A qualitative meta-synthesis examining the role of women in African American men's prostate cancer screening and treatment decision making. *Psycho-Oncology, 27*(3), 781–790. https://doi.org/10.1002/pon.4572

British Society for Rheumatology, & Health Quality Improvement Partnership. (2022). *The national early inflammatory arthritis audit (NAIAA)*.

Carretero, M. T., Calderón-Larrañaga, A., Poblador-Plou, B., & Prados-Torres, A. (2014). Primary health care use from the perspective of gender and morbidity burden. *BMC Women's Health, 14*(1), 145.

Courtenay, W. H. (2000). Constructions of masculinity and their influence on men's well-being: A theory of gender and health. *Social Science & Medicine, 50*(10), 1385–1401.

Doran, D., Williamson, S., Wright, K., & Beaver, K. (2018). "It's not just about prostate cancer, it's about being a gay man": A qualitative study of gay men's experiences of healthcare provision in the UK. *European Journal of Cancer Care, 27*(6), e12923. https://doi.org/10.1111/ecc.12923

Flurey, C., Morris, M., Pollock, J., Richards, P., Hughes, R., & Hewlett, S. (2014a). Fluctuating balances: A Q-methodology study of flare help-seeking behaviours and different experiences of daily life in Rheumatoid Arthritis. *BMC Musculoskeletal Disorders, 15*, 364.

Flurey, C., Morris, M., Richards, P., Hughes, R., & Hewlett, S. (2014b). "It's like a juggling act": Rheumatoid Arthritis patient perspectives on daily life and flare whilst on current treatment regimes. *Rheumatology, 53*(4), 696–703.

Hamed, S., Bradby, H., Ahlberg, B. M., & Thapar-Björkert, S. (2022). Racism in healthcare: A scoping review. *BMC Public Health, 22*(988). https://doi.org/10.1186/s12889-022-13122-y

Hunt, K., Adamson, J., Hewitt, C., & Nazareth, I. (2011). Do women consult more than men? A review of gender and consultation for back pain and headache. *Journal of Health Services Research and Policy, 16*(2), 108–117. https://doi.org/10.1258/JHSRP.2010.009131

Isano, S., Yohannes, T., Igihozo, G., Ndatinya, G. I., & Wong, R. (2023). A qualitative study to explore the healthcare-seeking experiences of men who have sex with men (MSM) and transgender women (TGW) in Rwanda. *BMC Health Services Research, 23*(1), 291. https://doi.org/10.1186/S12913-023-09286-X

Juel, K., & Christensen, K. (2008). Are men seeking medical advice too late? Contacts to general practitioners and hospital admissions in Denmark 2005. *Journal of Public Health, 30*(1), 111–113. https://doi.org/10.1093/pubmed/fdm087

Medina-Perucha, L., Yousaf, O., Hunter, M., & Grunfeld, E. (2017). Barriers to medical help-seeking among older men with prostate cancer. *Journal of Psychosocial Oncology, 35*(5), 531–543. https://doi.org/10.1080/07347332.2017.1312661

Newman, C. E., Gray, R., Brener, L., Jackson, L. C., Dillon, A., Saunders, V., Johnson, P., & Treloar, C. (2017). "I had a little bit of a bloke meltdown…But the next day, i was up": Understanding cancer experiences among aboriginal men. *Cancer Nursing, 40*(3), E1–E8. https://doi.org/10.1097/NCC.0000000000000399

O'Brien, R., Hunt, K., & Hart, G. (2005). 'It's caveman stuff, but that is to a certain extent how guys still operate': Men's accounts of masculinity and help seeking. *Social Science & Medicine, 61*(3), 503–516.

Oliffe, J., Rossnagel, E., Bottorff, J., Chambers, S., Caperchione, C., & Rice, S. (2020). Community-based men's health promotion programs: Eight lessons learnt and their caveats. *Health Promotion International, 35*, 1230–1240.

Paulson, M., Norberg, A., & Danielson, E. (2002). Men living with fibromyalgia-type pain: Experiences as patients in the Swedish health care system. *Journal of Advanced Nursing, 40*(1), 87–95. https://doi.org/10.1046/j.1365-2648.2002.02343.x

Quincey, K., Williamson, I., & Winstanley, S. (2016). 'Marginalised malignancies': A qualitative synthesis of men's accounts of living with breast cancer. *Social Science & Medicine, 149*, 17–25. https://doi.org/10.1016/J.SOCSCIMED.2015.11.032

Salifu, Y., Almack, K., & Caswell, G. (2023). 'Out of the frying pan into the fire': A qualitative study of the impact on masculinity for men living with advanced prostate cancer. *Palliative Care and Social Practice, 17*. https://doi.org/10.1177/26323524231176829/

Sharf, B., Stelljes, L., & Gordon, H. (2005). "A little bitty spot and I'm a big man": Patients' perspectives on refusing diagnosis or treatment for lung cancer. *Psycho-Oncology, 14*(8), 636–646. https://doi.org/10.1002/pon.885

Snell, G. E., Seage, C. H., & Mercer, J. (2023). A phenomenological study on the lived experience of men with chronic fatigue syndrome. *Journal of Health Psychology*. https://doi.org/10.1177/13591053231186385

Wagland, R., Nayoan, J., Matheson, L., Rivas, C., Brett, J., Collaco, N., Alexis, O., Gavin, A., Glaser, A. W., & Watson, E. (2019). Adjustment strategies amongst black African and black Caribbean men following treatment for prostate cancer: Findings from the Life After Prostate Cancer Diagnosis. *European Journal of Cancer Care, 29*(1). https://doi.org/10.1111/ecc.13183
Walker, A. Q., Blake, C. E., Moore, J. B., Wilcox, S., DuBois, K., Watkins, W., & K. (2022). Experiences of midlife and older African American men living with type 2 diabetes. *Ethnicity & Health, 27*(6), 1256–1270. https://doi.org/10.1080/13557858.2021.1910206
Wang, Y., Freemantle, N., Nazareth, I., & Hunt, K. (2014). Gender differences in survival and the use of primary care prior to diagnosis of three cancers: An analysis of routinely collected UK general practice data. *PLOS ONE, 9*(7), e101562.
White, A. (2007). Men and the problems of late diagnosis. In J. Heidelbaugh (Ed.), *Clinical men's health: Evidence in practice* (1st ed., pp. 31–43). Elsevier.
White, A., & Banks, I. (2009). Men and help seeking. In R. Kirby, C. Carson III, A. White, & M. Kirby (Eds.), *Men's health* (3rd ed., pp. 505–514). CRC Press.
White, A. K., & Johnson, M. (2000). Men making sense of their chest pain—niggles, doubts and denials. *Journal of Clinical Nursing, 9*(4), 534–541. https://doi.org/10.1046/j.1365-2702.2000.00413.x
Yaklin, S., Kim, M., & Social, J. H. (2022). African American men who become mental health advocates. *International Journal of Social Psychiatry, 68*(5), 981–990. https://doi.org/10.1177/00207640211012736
Yousaf, O., Grunfeld, E., & Hunter, M. (2013). A systematic review of the factors associated with delays in medical and psychological help-seeking among men. *Health Psychology Review, 9*(2), 264–276. https://doi.org/10.1080/17437199.2013.840954

CHAPTER 9

Support

"*I think you need an English language degree to express some of the feelings*"

Psychosocial is defined as the interrelation of individual thoughts and behaviours (psychological) and social relationships and structures (social). As I've discussed throughout this book, the psychosocial impact of long-term conditions includes concerns about prognosis and disease course, worries about long-term effects of treatment, body image, emotional difficulties, sex and intimacy, loss or reduction in activities due to the unpredictable nature of the condition, career prospects and loss of income, dealing with reliance on others, and the impact all of these can have on self-esteem and masculinity. Support for psychosocial issues includes but is not limited to self-management. It includes anything that supports patients within the social and psychological context of their condition. In the previous chapter we established men are not as bad as people think at seeking help and engaging with healthcare services for physical symptoms. However, it can be trickier to engage men in the psychosocial side of healthcare. This chapter will go some way towards addressing how services could be better tailored towards men.

C. Flurey, *Talking Men's Health*,
https://doi.org/10.1007/978-3-031-62593-0_9

9.1 Is Healthcare Feminised?

Men are often branded a ‘hard to reach’ group by clinicians, healthcare professionals, and researchers. However, the National Institute for Health and Care Research (NIHR) have redefined ‘hard to reach’ as ‘underserved’, which removes a victim-blaming element from this narrative and refocuses our attention on how services could be designed to better serve these groups (NIHR, 2022). It would be too simplistic to claim that health services serve women better than men, as the barriers women face in accessing appropriate care, diagnosis, or referrals are well documented (Getachew et al., 2020; Lockwood Estrin et al., 2021; Pierz et al., 2020). However, the psychosocial aspects of healthcare are often unintentionally designed in ways that suit the needs and preferences of women more than men.

From the moment you walk into a healthcare setting, there can be unintentional subtle indications of the space being feminised. Waiting rooms tend to be equipped with magazines most likely to be read by women (perhaps less so since the Covid pandemic and concerns of cross-contamination!), and the majority of front-facing staff (such as receptionists) are women. Nurses and allied healthcare professionals design and deliver the majority of holistic healthcare including services that address patients’ psychosocial support needs. In the UK over 80% of nurses are women, with similar proportions in the majority of countries globally (World Health Organisation, 2023). It should perhaps not be surprising that services predominantly designed and delivered by women appeal more to women. This is picked up on in the following quote from a man with chronic fatigue syndrome who highlights the services he’s aware of either are directly targeted at women or contain activities he considers feminised:

> *There are so many support groups out there for CFS which are targeted at mothers and often classes like yoga which I feel is female dominated. My male friends would definitely laugh at me for doing yoga anyway [laughs]. (Paul, 42yrs, chronic fatigue syndrome, White British)* (Snell et al., 2023)

There are often limited resources and funding for clinical teams to develop services tailored to the needs of different patient groups (with much of this work done above and beyond their work commitments). Additionally, healthcare professionals may not have been prompted to consider how men's needs may differ from women's. In fact, many healthcare professionals I speak to when presenting my work on men's health tell me they are aware far fewer men than women attend their services, but need advice on how to engage men or to develop services men would be interested in.

Women are more likely to take part in psychosocial research studies, which includes those that develop and test support interventions. Thus, the resulting intervention tends to reflect the needs and preferences of those who have taken part in these studies. This highlights the importance of ensuring that under-served groups are involved right from the beginning in studies to inform intervention development, and researchers may need to consider different recruitment approaches to engage these groups.

The feeling of healthcare being designed for women was particularly pronounced in conditions that affect women more than men. In breast cancer care, men consistently discuss encountering difficulties with there being no established way of caring and supporting men, particularly in relation to psychological support. This meant they were treated according to the methods prescribed for treating women, because the clinicians 'knew no other way'. This lack of acknowledgement of the different needs of men, or skills to address these, strengthened men's feelings of illegitimacy as breast cancer patients (Quincey et al., 2016).

In addition to ways that healthcare support services may be created through a feminised lens, men also describe a heteronormative approach to healthcare. Gay and bisexual men experience clinicians assuming they are heterosexual (e.g., asking about wives). This raised concerns about judgement from healthcare professionals if they disclosed their sexual orientation, which could further alienate them from healthcare services (Matheson et al., 2017). Gay and bisexual men with prostate cancer describe the information and advice they're given as geared towards heterosexual men. They found their clinicians didn't address their different needs—either due to being uninformed about safety concerns related to anal sex or making heterosexual assumptions. Gay and bisexual men with prostate cancer often tried to seek out this information elsewhere:

> *I'd read somewhere … that really men should wait about 3–4 weeks before resuming anal sex but I cannot find that literature anywhere on the NHS or Bupa [private health insurance company] I have scoured the internet. (gay man, prostate cancer, UK)* (Doran et al., 2018)

9.2 What Do Men Want from Their Clinical Team?

Throughout this book the ways the clinical team can support men in relation to specific issues (e.g., mental wellbeing, mortality, sex and intimacy) have been discussed. Drawing all of this together, men with long-term conditions valued the opportunity to build a relationship with their clinical team. This can build confidence and trust and break down some of the barriers created by the imbalance of a doctor-patient relationship, which can help regain some control. Men put trust in doctors who provide them with information and give them the opportunity to ask questions (Alexis & Worsley, 2018), and value those who get to know them well enough to pitch information at the right level. Men often want healthcare professionals to directly ask them about issues they find difficult to bring up themselves (e.g., sex and intimacy or mental wellbeing). Many men value healthcare professionals who take a direct, sometimes blunt, approach to telling them the course of their disease, and consequences for not self-managing or taking care of their health:

> *My doctor … he's straight up with me. He told me, 'Look, if you don't do this you are going to die. If you want to live, this is what you have to do, if you not going on dialysis, it's up to you.' He's … he's a real straight-up type of guy I like. 'Ok, I'm telling you what you got to do and that's it. … It is up to you.' So, he holds no punches. (type 2 diabetes, African American) (Walker et al.,* 2022)

Many men used dark humour to discuss their condition and appreciated it when their clinical team returned this as it helped them feel connected to them. However, this can be a difficult line to tread as a healthcare professional until sufficient rapport has been built up to know individual patients' humour. It shouldn't need to be said, but humour should never be used that even comes close to bordering on homophobic, racist, sexist, or in any way discriminatory. As the following quote demonstrates, offensive attempts at humour can shatter trust in a clinical relationship:

> *[I]t was incredibly difficult to talk to the doctor. … That was another reason why I didn't like the urologist because he made the joke, it [digital rectal examination] wouldn't be painful for me. … I can remember word for word, he said, 'well somebody like you, it won't make a lot of difference to somebody like you'. (gay man, prostate cancer, UK)* (Doran et al., 2018)

Finally, the question I'm most often asked by healthcare professionals is, "Do men prefer to be treated by men or women?" and the answer is, 'It depends'. Men are not an homogeneous group and as such have different preferences over clinician gender for different reasons. My own studies found no consistent answer, and this is born out throughout the long-term conditions literature. Some men preferred female clinicians finding them to have a gentler approach, or to be more sympathetic, or feeling more comfortable talking about emotions with them. Other men preferred male clinicians as they felt uncomfortable opening up to women about things they found embarrassing or emasculating. Some men had no preference at all, taking the attitude that 'a doctor's a doctor'. Overall, the approach taken to caring for and interacting with men far outweighed a healthcare professional's gender.

9.3 Should Support Be Male Only?

A systematic review of support across 40 randomised controlled trials (RCTs) of self-management support interventions in men and 20 RCTs where an analysis by sex was reported found insufficient evidence exists to make claims about whether men showed greater improvement in men-only or mixed-gender groups (Galdas et al., 2015). As with clinician gender, when we ask men whether they would prefer support to be mixed gender or male only they are fairly divided. This may be further complicated by there being different preferences depending on the topic that may be covered. In 2018 I conducted a survey study across 280 men with rheumatoid arthritis in England, and 62% of these men said they had no preference for whether support was male only or mixed gender. It's important to remember there may be an element of social desirability factoring into these responses with it being less socially acceptable to request male-only spaces (than female-only spaces). Additionally, men who took part in a survey didn't have the benefit of experiencing an all-male focus group, which prompted the men in this setting to consider ways in which the conversation may have been different if the group had been mixed. The following interaction from one of my focus groups with men with systemic sclerosis demonstrates these two differing opinions of male-only versus mixed-gender groups. Wade highlights that erectile dysfunction wouldn't have been as easy to talk about with women in the group, whilst Jacob takes the view that he would talk the same in front of anyone, and women may experience similar issues:

Wade *I think we would have felt more comfortable being like it is [male only focus group] because y'all are doctors [female facilitators]. You know what I'm saying, versus if we would have had half women in here and half men, I think the, the discussion of erectile dysfunction would not have been as lengthy, see what I'm getting at, it would have been very short-lived. I'm having a problem, the end, goodbye.*

CF *So is there an argument for male only groups?*

Jacob *I tell you the truth, I don't care who know about it, I gonna enjoy myself, you know, as long as my wife has me, I don't care who isn't going to like it, if she was sitting alongside of me, I say I can't do nothing, I can't. … I'm not ashamed of it, I think that's the truth, what you gon' to lie for. No need to lyin', you can't hide it, you know. … That's how I feel, it might, might be different for men, but some women probably don't be in the mood, you know.*

(Focus group with men with systemic sclerosis, USA)

Some studies have found men prefer mixed-gender groups (Cramer et al., 2014), whilst others discuss a desire for male-only environments for support. For some they saw male-only spaces as a safer environment to talk about themselves. Opening up can feel like demonstrating 'weakness', which they may be reluctant to do in front of women (Sattar et al., 2023). For some men having support within a dedicated men's group was more important than having the same condition, as this man with breast cancer explains:

> *So, I found the men's group. And even though I was the only one with breast cancer, I found it more comfortable and helpful. But I think that fact they had a specific men's group, it was very important in my journey and in my recovery. … I really found that women would react to me in a different way. (P-23, breast cancer, USA)* (Potter et al., 2023)

Research comparing interactions of friends and relatives in online forums for breast cancer (aimed at women) and prostate cancer (aimed at men) found that quantitatively women dominated both forums. Women were found to post frequently and to prioritise an emotional communication style (more commonly used by women) over an informational communication style (generally preferred by men). However, the men adapted their communication style to prioritise emotional communication to accommodate the norms of the opposite gender (Seale, 2006). Evidence from the obesity literature suggests that male-only groups are qualitatively different to mixed-gender groups with different levels of engagement, styles of language, and success (Robertson et al., 2014; Young et al., 2012). So, there may be an argument for male-only interventions to enable men to engage in the way they are most comfortable.

9.4 Involving Family in Support

Men have reported mixed preferences for spouse or partner involvement in support (Sattar et al., 2023). For men in relationships, long-term conditions were often managed together with their partners. For example, men often mentioned their partners being responsible for managing their diet ("*I eat whatever I'm given*" man with prostate cancer, (Hackshaw-Mcgeagh et al., 2017)), either for specific medical reasons such as diabetes control (Walker et al., 2022), to try and help them promote a healthier lifestyle, or in the hopes of helping control the disease ("*lots of cancer fighting vegetables*", man with lung cancer (Maersk et al., 2022)).

Many men throughout my focus groups highlighted the impact of their condition on their spouses or partners, and suggested including them in support interventions to provide them with their own support structures:

> *I think it's very important that we give our caregivers support in whatever way it be, if it be through study or through one on one psychiatric help, or just someone to talk to. I think that's very important 'cause I know my wife has been through hell and back. I had a lot of problems and, erm, she stood by my side and I know now, now I'm much better but it took me five years to get here. We went through some very hard times and she stood by me. (Wade, 61yrs, systemic sclerosis, White American)*

Men also sought empathy and understanding from their spouses or partners (Alexis & Worsley, 2018). So, to some the attraction of involving partners in support sessions was to provide a form of education to help their partners better understand them. The following interaction demonstrates this need to feel understood and highlights that men may not always find it easy to articulate their experiences to their partners and may value support in expressing this. It's also worth noting that Paul refers to this as a 'partner's day', indicating that male patient only support away from partners would also be welcome rather than partners being in regular attendance:

Paul	*I think you should have a partner's day as well. As I mentioned earlier, you know, the theme should be on us men, for helping us out, but definitely in any course or, or, or where you roll out these meetings, somewhere along the line there should be a partner's day where we can carefully educate them about scleroderma. So they come away from this hospital after two or three hours here, they think, 'oh …'*
Karim	*'I didn't realise that.'*
Paul	*'… I've got, I've got to look out for this in my man.'*
Emil	*They can appreciate the things you do.*
Karim	*Yeah.*
Paul	*'Cause they don't know, they don't know what we're going through because, I think you need an English language degree to express some of the feelings.*
	(Focus group with men with systemic sclerosis, UK)

An example of involving partners in support for men has been modelled in the 'Man-to-man and side-by-side' meetings for prostate cancer (Arrington et al., 2006). The design of these involves men and their partner (or carer/family member) meeting in one room together for the first hour to listen to a guest speaker (e.g., a urologist, oncologist, radiologist) with a question-and-answer session. This is followed by a snack break and then the men and their partners are split into separate rooms to discuss their own concerns (the men were also further divided into breakout groups depending on what they wanted to talk about, e.g., by treatment options they were considering). Researchers found the women's discussion focused primarily on their husbands rather than their own support needs, which may have been the product of facilitation style. Other issues related to communication were also highlighted, which I'll revisit later in this chapter in relation to social support (Sect. 9.7). However, the basic format of these groups has potential for providing both education and support for partners alongside men with long-term conditions, without partners encroaching on the men's support spaces.

It is important to note that not all men want their families involved in discussions related to their condition. Men sometimes mask the full impact of their condition to protect those close to them (discussed in Chaps. 3 and 7). Thus, there were certain elements of support that men did not want to talk about in front of family members they felt an urge to protect. Interviews with Black African and Black Caribbean men with prostate cancer found they were reluctant to share their experiences and management of cancer with their wives and partners. There was a cultural expectation that men were "*in the driving seat*" and these men didn't tend to communicate their concerns with their partners as they didn't want to be perceived as emotionally weak. As these men took on the management of their condition alone, this often meant they didn't recognise a need for their partners to have support (Bamidele et al., 2019).

This applies not only to group support, but clinicians should also be aware that if men are accompanied by a family member to their appointment, this may contribute to their reluctance to engage in emotional talk. It may be particularly important for healthcare professionals to advocate on behalf of younger men to have one-to-one time to enable them to talk about issues concerning them:

> *End of life conversations should happen but I don't want to ask about stuff in front of my mum, I don't want to upset her. (Duchenne muscular dystrophy, UK)* (Abbott et al., 2017)

Finally, it is important to note that not all men are in partnered relationships. While some unpartnered men found multiple sources of support through friends and family including adult children, others worried about burdening others and managed alone (Matheson et al., 2017). Unpartnered men may be more likely to rely on the doctor when making treatment decisions (Kazer et al., 2011). Thus, support that includes spouses or partners could be alienating for those men who potentially have the most to benefit from social support:

> *I have no close family at all. My friends don't want to be bothered. They don't want to hear about it. I have a paid caregiver who comes in four days a week, four and a half hours a day. (Thomas, 67yrs, prostate cancer, bisexual, White American).* (Capistrant et al., 2016)

9.5 Peer Support

In Chap. 7, I covered how men may be selective in who they open up to, and that the nature and amount of disclosure may change depending on who they are talking to. In my focus groups, men tended to value speaking to other men with the same condition, many of whom were having the opportunity to do this for the first time:

Robert	*Well, we've never had anybody to talk to about it before.*
David	*Don't ever have people to talk to so it makes a change.*
Robert	*No. Nobody else is interested, if they haven't got it they don't care do they?*
	(Focus group with men with rheumatoid arthritis)

The benefits of sharing experiences with other men with the same condition are widely recognised by men with long-term conditions (Galdas et al., 2014) and interventions that include a peer support component have been shown to have a positive impact on their quality of life (Galdas et al., 2015). Men with cancer found that disclosing their diagnosis to others helped them identify those who had similar experiences or knowledge to pass on and gained support in this way (Alexis & Worsley, 2018). Men in my focus groups and throughout the long-term conditions literature enjoyed being able to talk about their condition without the burden of having to explain their experiences as they felt understood. Shared experiences provide a feeling of validation, for example, men with systemic sclerosis were reassured to hear that other men in their group experience erectile dysfunction. This normalised their experiences in the context of their condition, meaning within this group they didn't have to worry about "*standing out from the herd*" (O'Brien et al., 2007).

Men valued learning from each other in my focus groups. They shared practical tips and emotional support. Those who were more newly diagnosed found value in speaking to others further along the journey and took comfort in see them coping both physically and emotionally. Some of my American participants with systemic sclerosis had been given the opportunity to take part in a peer mentoring programme and generally spoke positively about this. However, they noted that this could be difficult when the person they were paired with had much more progressed disease severity. This could lead to fears about their own disease progression, and feelings of guilt that they were accepting support from someone in a worse situation clinically.

Peer support can be particularly effective in supporting self-management and health behaviour change through enhancing access to information and resources, working together to problem solve, and adds an element of peer pressure or social obligation to stick to health goals (Lee et al., 2018). In Chap. 7, I mentioned gamifying self-management may be effective. Within this, healthy competition can be used in peer groups to further encourage healthy behaviour changes. Peer-led support and learning can be empowering as it hands back control to patients, rather than feeling they are being told what to do by an authority figure. When I asked participants who they would like to lead an intervention *"staff led but patient run" (Mike, 60yrs, rheumatoid arthritis, White British)* was suggested to enable patients to set the agenda, whilst staff would be helpful for making the practical arrangements or to answer questions. In men with depression, professionally led groups were more likely to be attended by men with higher mental health support needs, where these needs could be addressed indirectly (Cramer et al., 2014).

For many men, the shared experience of having the same condition provided sufficient similarity between them, and other social characteristics were less important. However, studies that attracted 'like-minded' men with shared interests (e.g., Football Fans in Training (Hunt et al., 2014), which will be discussed as a positive example of an intervention later in this chapter) highlighted that the more the men had in common with their peers the more accessible and acceptable they may find a peer support-based intervention (Galdas et al., 2014).

Many men with long-term conditions valued the experience of an 'insider' group feeling when amongst others who share the same condition. However, men from marginalised groups may still feel like 'outsiders' to these groups. For example, gay men with prostate cancer have found the structure and purpose of support groups unsuitable for their needs, feeling a sense of not belonging. They also found it uncomfortable to talk candidly about sexual issues in the presence of the other men's female partners (Doran et al., 2018). For these men having a condition in common is insufficient in spaces that don't make an effort to step out of heteronormative assumptions, and having sexuality in common for peer support may be more important than the specific cancer or condition:

> *I know some people had talked about how important it is to have a support group and if you go to a typical prostate support group it's all straight men and it's usually it's their wives that are talking. (Daniel, 70yrs, prostate cancer, gay, White American)* (Capistrant et al., 2016)

9.6 Creating a Trusted Environment: Setting

> *People say men don't talk, well that's bullshit, once they're in the right space you can't shut them up. (stakeholder working in men's health or community-based organisation, Australia)* (Sharp et al., 2022)

There is a wealth of evidence to show that if we create a safe, private, and trusted environment men will take part in support groups (Galdas et al., 2014). In considering what makes a trusted environment, we should first consider the setting. There is good evidence that meeting men where they are at, in spaces where they reside and frequent can be effective in promoting health engagement (Oliffe et al., 2020). This has been shown to be particularly successful in Barbershop settings, where health promotion interventions have improved uptake of cancer screening, blood pressure and blood sugar checks, along with strategies for optimising mental health, diet, and exercise. Placing health interventions in such a setting has the benefit of both convenience and being a safe and trusted environment with health information being taken from respected members of their community.

Whilst these setting are effective for preventative health measures, when it comes to long-term conditions their treating hospital often becomes a place that men frequent for their appointments. A survey study I conducted across England with men with rheumatoid arthritis found that of 280 men only 17% were interested in support being held in a location away from their hospital. Thus, it is possible that long-term conditions are distinct in that men may be more likely to trust and become familiar with their hospital, making it an appropriate setting for an intervention. Some men preferred to 'box' their condition with all their care delivered in the hospital rather than have a 'patient' identity encroach into settings where they reside. Additionally, men said they'd be motivated to attend support if they received an appointment letter (54%) or an invitation from their rheumatologist (67%) or specialist nurse (51%). This may indicate a need for legitimising self-management support as a key part of medical management, which delivery in the hospital setting also contributes to (Flurey et al., 2018a). However, it is also important to note that these findings reflect the views of those men who are engaged enough in their healthcare to take part in the study, and the 17% of men with rheumatoid arthritis who would prefer support delivered away from their hospital could reflect the very men who may benefit most from support.

9.7 Creating a Trusted Environment: Communication

Equally (or arguably more) important in creating a safe, private, and trusted environment is the communication style adopted. The importance of language with men's groups starts from the moment a group is named and advertised as this can send an important message to men about whether the group 'speaks' to them or not, which can have a marked impact on uptake and engagement. In thinking about language this should be understandable, accessible, inclusive of men from diverse backgrounds, and aligned with the target group's preferences and levels of health literacy (Galdas et al., 2023; Oliffe et al., 2020).

This focus on masculinised language is exemplified by the charity Talk Club (Talk Club, 2024) (discussed in Chap. 3), who brand themselves a male 'mental fitness' charity. This aligns with an evidence base that suggests avoiding medical labels such as 'mental health' can be more effective in engaging men (Oliffe et al., 2020). Talk Club use the term talking group instead of support group, their group facilitators are relabelled as 'coaches', and their social media marketing tells us "It's like the gym but for your mind". This language harnesses sport club metaphors to normalise taking care of mental health in the same way men would take care of their physical fitness. However, whilst masculinised language can be important for engagement, it is important to ensure that this doesn't extend into language that would have the potential to perpetuate negative masculine stereotypes such as "man up" (Galdas et al., 2023).

Communication styles and interactions are also crucial within the group setting for developing trusted environments. In my focus groups (as discussed in Chap. 1), I found men valued the discussion starting with 'safe' topics (such as comparing medication and physical symptoms) before moving onto topics that may involve revealing an element of vulnerability. Focusing discussion on functionality over feelings can facilitate a problem-solving dynamic, which can support rapport-building and make it easier for men to open up about sensitive topics (Galdas et al., 2014).

Men may need time to develop rapport to enable them to open up about emotional or sensitive issues, but as we've seen demonstrated in the quotes throughout this book given a trusted environment and permission to speak men will open up about a variety of issues. The role of providing permission to speak about emotional issues shouldn't be overlooked. Whilst group dynamics can facilitate engagement, they can also work to stifle it (Galdas et al., 2014). In this regard, a group facilitator can make or break the nature of the discussion.

In the 'Man-to-man and side-by-side' intervention for prostate cancer (previously discussed in Sect. 9.4), researchers found that the topics of discussion in either the men's or partner's groups rarely allowed for emotional expression. When emotional issues were raised, topic-turning was used by group members to steer away from topics perceived as uncomfortable and back towards a problem-solving focus. Little attention was given in group meetings to emotion, venting, confirmation of feelings, or consolation. With the importance of men being given explicit permission for emotional expression, it is possible that a real or perceived pressure to conform to a problem-focused group dynamic could be stifling men's ability to access support (Arrington et al., 2006).

One way of facilitating discussion about sensitive or emotional topics in a way that feels less loaded can be the use of humour. I've mentioned humour in a number of places throughout this book for the way some men choose to discuss their condition with friends or healthcare professionals, and this carries through to support groups. Humour can build rapport and connectedness between men in group settings, and can be used to introduce potentially sensitive topics in a 'safe' way that informally sought the group's permission to explore further (Oliffe et al., 2009):

> *I remember one of the fellows saying, well, heck, I'm 65 years old now, I've had lots of good sex in my life, I don't mind losing it now. … It's a very serious subject to most of us and it could be a pretty drab meeting if some humor wasn't injected. I don't think the attendance would be as good if you didn't have a little humor thrown in. (65yrs, prostate cancer, Canada)* (Oliffe et al., 2009)

As with every other time I've mentioned humour throughout this book it needs to be said that humour isn't universal. This has caused uncomfortable situations in support groups where men have felt their problems minimised or ridiculed with the use of humour they didn't feel part of (Oliffe et al., 2009). Nevertheless, humour can help men to stay positive and they can even laugh with each other about the consequences of their treatment (Branney et al., 2014). It's therefore important that group facilitators are mindful of this and can respond swiftly to defuse any well-meaning but misdirected attempts at humour.

Finally, it can be important to embrace silence to allow time for thought and self-reflection, or to help men focus on activity-based content (Oliffe et al., 2020). Men can also value being able to participate by listening to others without feeling pressure to actively contribute (Galdas et al., 2014).

9.8 The Need for a Purpose

Although the men seemed to value the opportunity to speak to each other in my focus groups, when I asked them if they would return to a similar group as part of their care, they were less enthusiastic (*"I don't know what I'd say [in a support group]. I'm here to help you [researcher]" Frank, rheumatoid arthritis* (Flurey et al., 2016b)). The research setting provided a clear purpose for the men to come together to talk about their experiences, and the opportunity for emotional expression was simply a welcome by-product of that. When I asked men what they would want from a support intervention, they were clear that they wanted this to be structured with a more concrete purpose than a talking group. I discussed in Chap. 7 how men were keen to develop expertise in their condition, so perhaps unsurprisingly when it came to support preferences, many of them wanted the opportunity to learn more about their condition, or how to manage it:

Pete *I'd like, if we're going to do those sort of things. I personally believe it should be a two way flow, so a bit of information on some of the latest developments and thinking from the clinical medical community ….*
James *Rather than a group, people that just come together and have a bit of a moan about their symptoms, if you're getting something, something structured out of it?*
(Focus group with men with systemic sclerosis, UK)

This need for support to have a clear purpose and address an unmet need is evident throughout the long-term conditions literature (Galdas et al., 2014). This purpose could involve an education component or physical activity, both of which have been shown to improve quality of life in men with long-term conditions (Galdas et al., 2015). However, it could also be an activity unrelated to their condition that has a shared purpose. Providing men with a shared activity works with the principle that men prefer 'side-by-side' rather than face-to-face support. Thus, creating spaces where men can provide shoulder-to-shoulder support for each other can be effective at creating a sense of belonging (Milligan et al., 2016). There seems to be a clear message from men that the support component shouldn't be the main focus of the activity but occur as a by-product of taking part in the shared activity (Sharp et al., 2022). Men's Sheds is perhaps one of the best and most well-known examples of this approach to providing shared activities leading to shoulder-to-shoulder support, which I'll discuss further below (Sect. 9.9).

9.9 Exemplar Intervention: Men's Sheds

Men's Sheds (Men's Sheds, 2024) is a flagship example of an intervention for men that creates a trusted environment for men to provide shoulder-to-shoulder support to each other through shared activities hosted in 'men's sheds' spaces. Men's Sheds was set up to address isolation and loneliness in older and retired men, providing shared spaces to engage in garden shed activities for men to 'connect, converse and create' together. The focus on activities occupies men and reduces the pressure to chat. This seems to create an environment in which men feel comfortable to chat without needing to acknowledge this is happening. A key design and delivery lesson from this initiative is that 'men connect by doing' (Oliffe et al., 2020):

> *I found that places like Men's Sheds, where it's never overt, there's a lot of debriefing, there's a lot of talking about feelings, although they wouldn't admit to that. But it's that sort of safety that men feel around other men often helps with their mental health stuff a lot. (Australia)* (Sharp et al., 2022)

Men's Sheds has been shown to decrease self-reported symptoms of depression in men. It promotes a sense of purpose through building relationships and sharing skills; it also encourages increased physical activity and cognitive skills. Men report feelings of pride and achievement, which positively impacts their self-esteem and self-worth (Culph et al., 2015):

> *It's given me a purpose to be here. That's what this place is. This place gives people a purpose. … It makes me feel like I'm worth something again. (Keith, depression, Australia)* (Culph et al., 2015)

Whilst Men's Sheds hasn't been created for, or directly applied as a support initiative for men with long-term conditions, there is great potential for it to be adapted for this purpose. The impact of long-term conditions on men's self-esteem and self-worth was discussed in Chap. 2, and the shared purpose and pride in working together to create something could have clear benefits in helping to restore this. I discussed in Chap. 7 that many men make their own tools and devices to help them adjust and adapt to disability with a long-term condition. A Men's Sheds set up with a focus on shared problem-solving and creation of adaptive tools and devices could be a rewarding initiative that may work to engage men.

The practical focus of Men's Sheds tends to be focused on making or working on something that would traditionally be done in a shed, but we don't have to be limited to this. For example, Men's Pie Club (Men's Pie Club, 2024) is a Newcastle-based social enterprise that uses similar principles, but the shared activity is making pies. Each week men decide on the filling for the next week together, and then come together to make pies. Men's Sheds lays the groundwork for finding a shared interest, passion, or activity and through this, enabling men to find meaning, connection, and support.

9.10 Exemplar Intervention: Football Fans in Training

Football Fans in Training (FFIT) is another often-cited example of an intervention for men. This is a physical activity intervention aimed at tackling obesity in men, which has been particularly lauded for its gender-sensitised approach in every aspect of delivery. Delivered in 13 professional football clubs, the programme was gender-sensitised for context (football clubs and men-only groups), content (focusing on the science of weight loss presented simply, discussion of alcohol and its potential role in weight management, and branding with club insignia), and style of delivery (participative and peer-supported, with male 'banter' encouraged to help with discussion of sensitive subjects). FFIT was free of charge, with 90-minute sessions every week for 12 weeks at the club's home stadium. There was a balance of classroom and physical activity sessions, which was weighted more towards physical activity as the men's fitness improved. Participants were also taught behavioural change techniques for physical activity and diet (e.g., self-monitoring, goal setting). This was not only popular but effective. They found significant differences in favour of the intervention for weight loss, body fat percentage, blood pressure, physical activity levels, consumption of alcohol, fats and sugars, and improved psychological and quality of life outcomes (Hunt et al., 2014). Additionally, improvements were maintained (with some attrition) 3.5 years later, demonstrating the value of this gendered approach to supporting men (Gray et al., 2018).

Looking beyond FFIT to other physical activity interventions, men with prostate cancer, who had experienced a 12-week recreational football training intervention, discussed how the social component embodied in team sports (i.e., football) was essential for their perception of exercise as meaningful and relevant. They also found the competitive and team element provided a sense of purpose and fun, which encouraged them to participate in a way that simply going for a run wouldn't (Bruun et al., 2014). This use of competitiveness as motivation further validates the suggestion that gamifying self-management may be effective for men (see Chap. 7). Mutual support and camaraderie with peers were key benefits of physical activity interventions for men with prostate cancer, providing them with the shared purpose needed to facilitate this (Sattar et al., 2023).

Physically demanding activities such as football may be more appropriate for some long-term conditions than others. For example, men with rheumatic diseases would need to be careful not to cause additional joint damage through the impact on their joints. Low-impact physical activity such as walking football could be considered, which would still retain the element of competition and teamwork.

When it comes to sports and physical activity one size doesn't fit all, and it's important to avoid lazy stereotypes of assuming all men would be drawn towards a football-themed intervention. When FFIT was delivered in European countries, recruitment strategies proved more successful in Portugal and the UK than the Netherlands and Norway, where there is perhaps less of a football-focused culture (Bunn et al., 2023). Nevertheless, men may be more drawn to physical activity that aligns with their view of masculinity as 'doing health' can represent a form of 'doing gender' (Robertson, 2007).

9.11 Summary

Men are often under-served when it comes to healthcare, with support services often unintentionally designed in ways that suit the needs and preferences of women. Men are not an homogeneous group so when it comes to support there is no single way that will work for all men. Thus, there are mixed views on whether support should be male only, and whether (and to what extent) family should be involved in support. Overall, men do value peer support, where they can feel part of an 'insider' group to share experiences without having to explain themselves. Men from marginalised groups may still feel like 'outsiders' to these groups and so may value support amongst those with a shared identity over having the same condition. Men will join groups, and they will open up when provided with a safe, private, trusted environment with the space to express themselves in a language they feel comfortable with. Support services for men work best if they have a clear shared purpose with emotional expression and support occurring as a by-product of this. Much can be learnt from existing interventions such as Men's Sheds and Football Fans in Training in providing a model for effective support for men that can be built on and tailored to men with long-term conditions.

References

Abbott, D., Prescott, H., Forbes, K., Fraser, J., & Majumdar, A. (2017). Men with Duchenne muscular dystrophy and end of life planning. *Neuromuscular Disorders, 27*(1), 38–44.

Alexis, O., & Worsley, A. J. (2018). A meta-synthesis of qualitative studies exploring men's sense of masculinity post-prostate cancer treatment. *Cancer Nursing, 41*(4), 298–310. https://doi.org/10.1097/NCC.0000000000000509

Arrington, M. I., Grant, C. H., & Vanderford, M. L. (2006). Man to man and side by side, they cope with prostate cancer: Self-help and social support. *Journal of Psychosocial Oncology, 23*(4), 81–102.

Bamidele, O., McGarvey, H., Lagan, B. M., Parahoo, K., Chinegwundoh, M. B. E., & F., & McCaughan, E. (2019). "Man in the driving seat": A grounded theory study of the psychosocial experiences of Black African and Black Caribbean men treated for prostate cancer and their partners. *Psycho-Oncology, 28*(8), 1712–1720. https://doi.org/10.1002/PON.5150

Branney, P., Witty, K., Braybrook, D., Bullen, K., White, A., & Eardley, I. (2014). Masculinities, humour and care for penile cancer: A qualitative study. *The Journal of Advanced Nursing, 70*(9), 2051–2060. https://doi.org/10.1111/jan.12363

Bruun, D. M., Krustrup, P., Hornstrup, T., Uth, J., Brasso, K., Rørth, M., Christensen, J. F., & Midtgaard, J. (2014). "All boys and men can play football": A qualitative investigation of recreational football in prostate cancer patients. *Scandinavian Journal of Medicine & Science in Sports, 24*(SUPPL.1), 113–121. https://doi.org/10.1111/sms.12193

Bunn, C., Palmer, V., Chng, N. R., Andersen, E., Gray, C. M., & Hunt, … Wyke, S. (2023). How European Fans in Training (EuroFIT), a lifestyle change program for men delivered in football clubs, achieved its effect: A mixed methods process evaluation embedded in a randomised controlled trial. *BMC Public Health, 23*(1). https://doi.org/10.1186/S12889-023-15419-Y

Capistrant, B. D., Torres, B., Merengwa, E., West, W. G., Mitteldorf, D., & Rosser, B. R. S. (2016). Caregiving and social support for gay and bisexual men with prostate cancer. *Psycho-Oncology, 25*(11), 1329–1336. https://doi.org/10.1002/pon.4249

Cramer, H., Horwood, J., Payne, S., Araya, R., Lester, H., & Salisbury, C. (2014). Do depressed and anxious men do groups? What works and what are the barriers to help-seeking? *Primary Health Care Research & Development, 15*(3), 287–301.

Culph, J., Wilson, N., Cordier, R., & Stancliffe, R. (2015). Men's Sheds and the experience of depression in older Australian men. *Australian Occupational Therapy Journal, 62*(5), 306–315. https://doi.org/10.1111/1440-1630.12190

Doran, D., Williamson, S., Wright, K., & Beaver, K. (2018). "It's not just about prostate cancer, it's about being a gay man": A qualitative study of gay men's experiences of healthcare provision in the UK. *European Journal of Cancer Care, 27*(6), e12923. https://doi.org/10.1111/ecc.12923

Flurey, C., Hewlett, S., Rodham, K., White, A., Noddings, R., & Kirwan, J. (2016b). "You obviously just have to put on a brave face": A qualitative study of the experiences and coping styles of men with rheumatoid arthritis. *Arthritis Care & Research, 69*(3), 330–337.

Flurey, C., Hewlett, S., Rodham, K., White, A., Noddings, R., & Kirwan, J. R. (2018a). Coping strategies, psychological impact and support preferences of men with rheumatoid arthritis: A multicentre survey. *Arthritis Care & Research, 70*(6), 851–860.

Galdas, P., Darwin, Z., Kidd, L., Blickem, C., McPherson, K., Hunt, K., Bower, P., Gilbody, S., & Richardson, G. (2014). The accessibility and acceptability of self-management support interventions for men with long term conditions: A systematic review and meta-synthesis of qualitative studies. *BMC Public Health, 14*(1), 1230.

Galdas, P., Fell, J., Bower, P., Kidd, L., Blickem, C., McPherson, K., Hunt, K., Gilbody, S., & Richardson, G. (2015). The effectiveness of self-management support interventions for men with long-term conditions: A systematic review and meta-analysis. *BMJ Open, 5*(e006620). https://doi.org/10.1136/bmjopen-2014-006620

Galdas, P. M., Seidler, Z. E., & Oliffe, J. L. (2023). Designing men's health programs: The 5C Framework. *American Journal of Men's Health, 17*(4). https://doi.org/10.1177/15579883231186463

Getachew, S., Tesfaw, A., Kaba, M., Wienke, A., Taylor, L., Kantelhardt, E. J., & Addissie, A. (2020). Perceived barriers to early diagnosis of breast Cancer in south and southwestern Ethiopia: A qualitative study. *BMC Women's Health, 20*(1). https://doi.org/10.1186/S12905-020-00909-7

Gray, C. M., Wyke, S., Zhang, R., Anderson, A. S., Barry, S., Brennan, G., Briggs, A., Boyer, N., Bunn, C., Donnachie, C., Grieve, E., Kohli-Lynch, C., Lloyd, S., Mcconnachie, A., Mccowan, C., Mclean, A., Mutrie, N., & Hunt, K. (2018). Long-term weight loss following a randomised controlled trial of a weight management programme for men delivered through professional football clubs: The Football Fans in Training follow-up study. *Public Health Research, 6*(9). https://doi.org/10.3310/phr06090

Hackshaw-Mcgeagh, L. E., Sutton, E., Persad, R., Aning, J., Bahl, A., Koupparis, A., Millett, C., Martin, R. M., & Lane, J. A. (2017). Acceptability of dietary and physical activity lifestyle modification for men following radiotherapy or radical prostatectomy for localised prostate cancer: A qualitative investigation. *BMC Urology, 17*(1), 1–11. https://doi.org/10.1186/S12894-017-0284-5

Hunt, K., Wyke, S., Gray, C. M., Anderson, A. S., Brady, A., Bunn, C., Donnan, P. T., Fenwick, E., Grieve, E., & Leishman, J. (2014). A gender-sensitised weight loss and healthy living programme for overweight and obese men delivered by Scottish Premier League football clubs (FFIT): A pragmatic randomised controlled trial. *The Lancet, 383*(9924), 1211–1221.

Kazer, M. W., Harden, J., Burke, M., Sanda, M. G., Hardy, J., & Bailey, D. E. (2011). The experiences of unpartnered men with prostate cancer: A qualitative analysis. *Journal of Cancer Survivorship, 5*(2), 132–141. https://doi.org/10.1007/S11764-010-0157-3

Lee, S., Schorr, E., Hadidi, N. N., Kelley, R., Treat-Jacobson, D., & Lindquist, R. (2018). Power of peer support to change health behavior to reduce risks for heart disease and stroke for African American men in a faith-based community. *Journal of Racial and Ethnic Health Disparities, 5*(5), 1107–1116. https://doi.org/10.1007/S40615-018-0460-7

Lockwood Estrin, G., Milner, V., Spain, D., Happé, F., & Colvert, E. (2021). Barriers to Autism Spectrum Disorder diagnosis for young women and girls: A systematic review. *Review Journal of Autism and Developmental Disorders, 8*(4), 454–470. https://doi.org/10.1007/S40489-020-00225-8

Maersk, J., Larsen, J., Rosted, E., & Lindahl-Jacobsen, L. (2022). "When I can ride my bike, I think, am I at all as sick as they say?": An exploration of how men with advanced lung cancer form illness perceptions in everyday life. *European Journal of Cancer Care, 31*(6), e13751. https://doi.org/10.1111/ecc.13751

Matheson, L., Watson, E., Nayoan, J., Wagland, R., Glaser, A., Gavin, A., Wright, P., & Rivas, C. (2017). A qualitative metasynthesis exploring the impact of prostate cancer and its management on younger, unpartnered and gay men. *European Journal of Cancer Care, 26*(6). https://doi.org/10.1111/ecc.12676

Men's Pie Club. (2024). *Men's Pie Club.* https://www.menspieclub.co.uk/about

Men's Sheds. (2024). *Men's Sheds.* https://menssheds.org.uk/

Milligan, C., Neary, D., Payne, S., Hanratty, B., Irwin, P., & Dowrick, C. (2016). Older men and social activity: A scoping review of Men's Sheds and other gendered interventions. *Ageing and Society, 36*(5), 895–923. https://doi.org/10.1017/S0144686X14001524

NIHR. (2022, January). *Improving inclusion of under-served groups in clinical research: Guidance from INCLUDE project.* https://www.NIHR.ac.UK/

documents/improving-Inclusion-of-under-served-groups-in-clinical-research-guidance-from-include-project/25435.

O'Brien, R., Hart, G. J., & Hunt, K. (2007). "Standing out from the herd": Men renegotiating masculinity in relation to their experience of illness. *International Journal of Men's Health, 6*(3), 178–200.

Oliffe, J., Rossnagel, E., Bottorff, J., Chambers, S., Caperchione, C., & Rice, S. (2020). Community-based men's health promotion programs: Eight lessons learnt and their caveats. *Health Promotion International, 35*, 1230–1240.

Oliffe, J. L., Ogrodniczuk, J., Bottorff, J. L., Hislop, T. G., & Halpin, M. (2009). Connecting humor, health, and masculinities at prostate cancer support groups. *Psycho-Oncology, 18*(9), 916–926. https://doi.org/10.1002/pon.1415

Pierz, A. J., Randall, T. C., Castle, P. E., Adedimeji, A., Ingabire, C., Kubwimana, G., Uwinkindi, F., Hagenimana, M., Businge, L., Musabyimana, F., Munyaneza, A., & Murenzi, G. (2020). A scoping review: Facilitators and barriers of cervical cancer screening and early diagnosis of breast cancer in Sub-Saharan African health settings. *Gynecologic Oncology Reports, 33*, 100605. https://doi.org/10.1016/J.GORE.2020.100605

Potter, A. M., Bentz, B., Crue, L., Leiby, S., Bashi, S., Maguire, K., Meyers, J., & Mieczkowski, K. (2023). Men's lived experiences of breast cancer and changes in occupation. *Occupational Therapy International.* https://doi.org/10.1155/2023/9641922

Quincey, K., Williamson, I., & Winstanley, S. (2016). 'Marginalised malignancies': A qualitative synthesis of men's accounts of living with breast cancer. *Social Science & Medicine, 149*, 17–25. https://doi.org/10.1016/J.SOCSCIMED.2015.11.032

Robertson, C., Archibald, D., Avenell, A., Douglas, F., Hoddinott, P., Boyers, D., Stewart, F., Boachie, C., Fioratou, E., & Wilkins, D. (2014). Systematic reviews of and integrated report on the quantitative, qualitative and economic evidence base for the management of obesity in men. *Health Technology Assessment, 18*(35), 1–458.

Robertson, S. (2007). *Understanding men and health: Masculinities, identity and well-being*. Open University Press.

Sattar, S., Haase, K., Bradley, C., Papadopoulos, E., Kuster, S., Mina, D., Tippe, M., Kaur, A., Campbell, D., Joshua, A., Rediger, C., Souied, O., & Alibhai, S. (2023). Barriers and facilitators related to undertaking physical activities among men with prostate cancer: A scoping review. *Prostate Cancer and Prostatic Diseases, 24*, 1007–1027.

Seale, C. (2006). Gender accommodation in online cancer support groups. *Health, 10*(3), 345–360. https://doi.org/10.1177/1363459306064495

Sharp, P., Bottorff, J. L., Rice, S., Oliffe, J. L., Schulenkorf, N., Impellizzeri, F., & Caperchione, C. M. (2022). "People say men don't talk, well that's bullshit": A focus group study exploring challenges and opportunities for men's mental health promotion. *PLOS ONE, 17*(1), e0261997. https://doi.org/10.1371/JOURNAL.PONE.0261997

Snell, G. E., Seage, C. H., & Mercer, J. (2023). A phenomenological study on the lived experience of men with chronic fatigue syndrome. *Journal of Health Psychology.* https://doi.org/10.1177/13591053231186385

Talk Club. (2024). *Talk Club.* https://talkclub.org/

Walker, A. Q., Blake, C. E., Moore, J. B., Wilcox, S., DuBois, K., Watkins, W., & K. (2022). Experiences of midlife and older African American men living with type 2 diabetes. *Ethnicity & Health, 27*(6), 1256–1270. https://doi.org/10.1080/13557858.2021.1910206

World Health Organisation. (2023). *Nurses by sex (%).* https://www.WHO.int/data/GHO/data/indicators/indicator-details/GHO/nurses-by-sex-(-)

Young, M. D., Morgan, P. J., Plotnikoff, R. C., Callister, R., & Collins, C. E. (2012). Effectiveness of male-only weight loss and weight loss maintenance interventions: A systematic review with meta-analysis. *Obesity Reviews, 13*(5), 393–408.

CHAPTER 10

Men Talking in Metaphors

"A computer virus, it's got an endless loop that won't stop"

The term 'metaphor' has two different uses, both originating with Aristotle in 4c BC. A metaphor is a literary figure of speech that uses an image, story, or tangible thing to represent a less tangible or intangible concept or quality. The term 'metaphor' can also be used more broadly to encompass any rhetorical figures of speech that achieve their effects through association, comparison, or resemblance. Thus, in this broader definition, simile, hyperbole, metonymy, and antithesis can also be considered types of metaphor (McArthur, 1992). In this chapter, I'll take as many liberties with 'metaphor' as Alanis Morrisette did with 'ironic' in the 1990s and adopt the broader of the two definitions. This will allow me to discuss the various types of language men use to talk about health rather than being limited to a strict definition of metaphor.

10.1 Why Metaphors Matter

It has been argued that a person's conceptual system, which governs their thoughts and structures their perception of the world, is largely metaphorical (Lakoff & Johnson, 1980). Since communication is based on the same conceptual system used in thinking and acting, the language we use can provide evidence for what that conceptual system might be. Thus, in theory, metaphors may create social realities and can be a guide for future

C. Flurey, *Talking Men's Health*,
https://doi.org/10.1007/978-3-031-62593-0_10

actions that fit the metaphor, reinforcing its power and making the experience coherent. A political example of this is "*War on Terror*", a metaphor that generated an '*enemy*', and a '*threat to national security*'. This metaphor introduced the concept that the intangible concept of '*terror*' could be personified as an enemy, which lead to policy change and political action. Thus, a metaphor can begin to define its own reality and can play a central role in the construction of social and political reality (Lakoff & Johnson, 1980). Exploring how men use metaphors may provide useful insights into how they conceptualise living with a long-term condition.

From a psychotherapy perspective, some argue that metaphors allow us to get in touch with our unconscious feelings and concerns (Modell, 2005). In children, fantasising and storytelling can be a way of making sense of the world around them (Bettelheim, 2010), and it's possible that the use of metaphors in adults could be an extension of this creative way of sense-making. If metaphors are the "*language of the soul [and] the discourse of the inner world*" (Wurmser, 2011) then looking at the metaphors used by men in relation to health has the potential to uncover a deeper, more meaningful understanding of their individual experiences and perceptions of living with a long-term condition.

In a healthcare setting, metaphors can assist both healthcare professionals and the patient. For the healthcare professional, metaphors can be a time-efficient tool for helping patients understand biologic processes (Arroliga et al., 2002). For patients, metaphors can increase empowerment (Harpham, 2010) and improve comprehension and retention of health and illness explanations (Whaley, 2000). Metaphors can also be used by family members to help make sense of their loved one's experience (Mastergeorge, 1999). The shared language of metaphors can aid the therapeutic relationship by providing a shared understanding of clinical reality (Reisfield & Wilson, 2004).

Children with asthma have described their condition as "*a boa constrictor squeezing the life out of you*"; a "*troll [that] sleeps all day in the dark ... until I wake him up by the activities I do, [then] he climbs up the ladder to tell the air it has to pay to come into my chest*", or "*[a] guardian angel [that] helps me to be good. However, if I mess up, I will get into trouble. My guardian angel does not protect me and can even take the air away*" (Peterson & Sterling, 2009). These metaphors provide a powerful insight into the way in which these children perceive the experience of asthma and make sense of the cause.

Metaphors are also used in both family therapy and cognitive behavioural therapy (CBT). Family therapy uses a technique called the animal attribution story-telling technique (AASTT), which is used to engage children with behavioural disorders. AASTT involves asking children to assign animals to each of their family members and tell a story that includes all the animals. This technique is seen as fun, non-threatening, and encourages participation. It provides the clinician with material that begins to explain the relationships within the family and provides a 'safe' way of discussing this (Arad, 2004). Metaphors have been used in CBT as a tool to assist with information processing or to provide a model for the change that a patient is trying to undertake (Otto, 2000).

Not everyone is a fan of metaphors being used in relation to illness. Susan Sontag wished to eliminate metaphors from the cancer discourse, believing that removing the symbolic associations would enable patients to see cancer as a biological phenomenon rather than a social or moral one (Clow, 2001). Later in this chapter when I cover the 'illness as war' metaphor I will discuss how metaphors can have negative connotations. However, throughout this chapter there are also examples of metaphors being used in ways that may facilitate understanding and coping with a long-term condition.

It can be argued that metaphors are culturally specific and may therefore not be universally understood, but it is precisely this culturally specific nature that makes them valuable in emphasising the degree of emotion in a situation (Richardson & Grose, 2009) and in connecting with patients in terminology that means something to them. The use of metaphors has been shown to be used in many health conditions as a way of grasping emotionally difficult concepts and of finding meaning in intangible thoughts and ideas (Lakoff & Johnson, 1980).

However, it is important to note that what for some may be commonly used and easily understood metaphors, may still be alien concepts to others and can hamper communication or even damage relationships through misunderstanding. The following quote from Alan demonstrates how a healthcare professional's well-meaning use of metaphor to facilitate coping and acceptance was interpreted almost literally and contributed to a negative experience of the understanding of his condition:

Alan *She [nurse] said 'treat this like a death'. I said, 'What do you mean a death?' She said you had to treat it as a death because it's something you're always going to have, and it put me right off. I said to my wife,*

'What's going on here? She said, 'They've got to treat this disease like a death,' you know. She did honestly, and I couldn't believe what was being said to me there.

CF *Do you think she meant bereavement?*

Alan *Oh yeah probably did mean that, but it didn't make me feel any better. (64yrs, rheumatoid arthritis, White British)*

10.2 Illness as War

The most common metaphors I've seen highlighted by authors throughout the literature relating to men with long-term conditions are war or battle metaphors. Men are often said to use 'fighting' talk when they discuss living with a long-term condition. The condition is described as a battle that can be won or lost: *"it hits you", "you battle through it", "I tried to fight it", "you're fighting a losing battle", "you can't beat it"*. This could indicate that patients attempt to counter-act the powerlessness they feel due to long-term conditions with a power-based metaphor. This is commonly interpreted as a particularly male approach to dealing with or speaking about illness—painting themselves as wounded warriors in a challenging fight against an undefeatable enemy. Battle talk reflects the importance that men can place on strength and courage in defining masculinity (Connell & Messerschmidt, 2005) and can easily be related to traditionally masculine images of men fighting at war (Snell et al., 2023).

However, for both patients and clinicians war is a dominant metaphor for illness, particularly within the cancer discourse (Reisfield & Wilson, 2004). This made me wonder if this was a particularly male way of speaking about illness, or whether we just expect to see this in men's narratives and therefore notice it more. So, I actively searched for battle metaphors throughout my previous interview transcripts with women with rheumatoid arthritis and found they seem to use this metaphor just as much as men. They use the same terminology with similar implications of a battle that they try to fight and don't always win:

> *I'd say the fatigue is the one thing that really gets you. And there's no way of trying to fight through that one, you know, with the pain and the swelling and everything else, you can fight through it, you can take the tablets, but with the fatigue, there's nothing, you've just got to go with it. (Chloe, 42yrs, rheumatoid arthritis, White British)*

I have to feel really really, that it's beaten me to go to bed actually. (Linda, 52yrs, rheumatoid arthritis, White British)

This way of speaking about illness, personified as an external force that needs to be fought against, has been widely popularised by the media and is commonly used even by patient-focused charities. The public are asked to: "*Play your part and together we will beat cancer*" (Cancer Research UK, 2023), "*Stand up to cancer*" (Stand up to cancer, 2023), "*Know diabetes, Fight diabetes*" (Diabetes UK, 2023). Thus, despite war metaphors being inherently masculine, power-based, paternalistic, and violent (Mitchell et al., 2003) the popularised use of these makes it difficult to draw conclusions about the meaning of these to men themselves. Similar terms can be found in the media in relation to the common cold, which of course doesn't have the same impact on people's lives as a long-term condition. Thus, it seems that illness as war or battle is now quite widely used for even minor illness, which may have removed some of the power that these fighting terms once carried. Thus, the use of these by men in relation to a long-term condition could easily represent language adopted from common usage rather than an underlying desire by men to be seen to be strong and courageous in the face of illness.

Whilst widely recognised, the metaphor of illness as war can be problematic when stretched beyond descriptions of the impact of a condition. For some patients conflict and fighting are not the preferred ways of coping with illness (Bowker, 1996; Hawkins, 1999). Labels such as 'brave' and 'strong' can create unnecessary implied pressure to wear a stoic mask. For patients living with a life-limiting condition, the suggestion of a battle that can be lost or won can unfairly imply death may be the result of failing to fight hard enough.

10.3 The Body as Both Hero and Villain

Whilst war as a metaphor for illness personifies the condition itself as an external force that needs to be defeated, men also talked in terms of the issue coming from inside them. One man described breast cancer as "*the enemy within*" and self-management and treatment was expressed as having to "*engage with the enemy*" (Quincey et al., 2016). Whilst there is much overlap in the language of illness as war, there is a subtle difference in the way the body itself can be personified as something that can be fought or that can provide defence.

John discusses the complicated nature of living with an auto-immune condition whereby the body's immune system attacking itself causes the symptoms he experiences. He talks about his immune system as 'destroying' or 'killing' his body. In thinking aloud how best to manage the condition, he splits his immune system from the rest of his body, conceptualising them as two different competing 'sides' and expresses a difficulty in knowing which 'side' to choose:

> *I me-mean when your body's fighting your body, who do you root for? I mean whi-which side are you on, you don't what side do you pick, do you go, I've got to get super strong, super healthy so I can improve my immune system so it can destroy the rest of my body. Or should I try to starve my immune system so it won't kill the rest of my body, I mean you don't know which side you're on and to route for. (John, 61yrs, systemic sclerosis, White American)*

The body was not only personified as an enemy but could also be a hero defending them against the condition. Here a man with lung cancer personifies the cells inside his body as soldiers fighting cancer:

> *Of course, I am never going to give up. I know that I am going to get through this. I have these 'soldiers' [cells combating cancer] inside me, and they will win this war. (George, 54yrs, lung cancer, Denmark)* (Maersk et al., 2022)

This dividing of the body as separate from the self resonates with the psychic defence mechanism of 'splitting' (Klein, 1952), which is the separation of one item into two, so that they can be handled separately. It has been suggested that when a person holds two thoughts in their mind that are contradictory or uncomfortable, the person will cognitively separate them, not thinking of the separate thoughts at the same time. This is a process of 'psychic economy' whereby a complex situation is simplified by separation rather than resolution. In this way, people can split 'whole objects' (a whole person) into 'part objects' (e.g., the body and the mind), which can be 'good' or 'bad'. The 'good part objects' can then be retained, loved, and admired whilst the 'bad part object' is externalised and attacked or repressed. This allows people to like themselves, while still recognising some unlikeable qualities. Or in the case of living with a long-term condition, bodies themselves can become the 'good' or 'bad' objects, enabling men to retain their sense of self and masculinity within a body that doesn't behave as desired.

10.4 Wounded Warriors

Still related to the metaphor of illness as a battle, men sometimes described themselves as 'warriors' or even 'gladiator' in relation to living with a long-term condition (Quaglia, 2020). However, the illness experience could be a reminder of their mortality and challenged their ability to embody masculine ideals. This was often expressed in metaphors of the men being wounded warriors, fallen heroes, or a loss of (imagined) superpowers:

> *All of a sudden you wake up one morning, oh my goodness me, I'm not invincible, I'm not a reasonably healthy 52 year old bloke, I, I could be dead in three years' time. (Paul, 52yrs, systemic sclerosis, White British)*

> *Yeah. It's made a big difference. You can get on and do things … but not think you're Superman where you're going to muck yourself up. (Ron, 60yrs, rheumatoid arthritis, White British)*

Beyond no longer holding superhero qualities, some men conjured up horror imagery, relating themselves to monsters or creatures. This sometimes seems to have been used to lighten discussion related to altered physical appearance, which may stem from societal expectations that men are meant to be less bothered about how they look. However, this also indicates men's dissatisfaction with their altered appearance and relationship with their masculine identity. It is of note that the creatures they compare themselves to are not strong and fierce monsters; instead they represent death and decay, highlighting the loss of a strong, healthy appearance:

> *They, they let me come into work late, they put up with the fact that I refused to stop working which was quite nice [laughs] really, 'cause there's this creature out of a morgue wandering in at them [laughs]. (Mark, systemic sclerosis, White British)*

> *I looked like sort of the living dead, a sort of zombie from a movie with drawn skin, just sort of a bony horrible creature. I think people were shocked when they saw me. (P4, oesophageal cancer, White British)* (Stapleton & Pattison, 2014)

10.5 Illness as an Unpredictable Predator: Loss of Power and Control

A feeling of loss of power and control has been highlighted throughout this book as a key impact on men living with a long-term condition. This can also be seen through both the metaphors that have naturally occurred throughout men's narratives, and in men who I asked to describe their condition as an animal.

In an attempt to capture either the most important aspects of living with rheumatoid arthritis or those concepts that patients may find difficult to express in a general conversation, in interviews with both men and women with rheumatoid arthritis I asked participants: "*If your rheumatoid arthritis were an animal, what animal would it be?*". The prompt of an animal was chosen as animals are universally relevant—animals as symbols exist in all cultures; they are in sayings such as '*the early bird catches the worm*' and in myths, fairy tales, and fables. Asking patients to relate to an animal invites them to consider its specific characteristics and symbolic meaning, which allows for a range of experiences, emotions, and perceptions to be acknowledged in a single animal image (Arad, 2004).

Participants were often drawn to deadly, dangerous, or vicious predatory animals to characterise rheumatoid arthritis, and they often represented the unpredictability and uncertainty of the condition:

> *Yeah you have got snakes because they are horrible and sinister and sneaky and you know you don't know when they are going to come and attack you or anything like this. (James, 47yrs, rheumatoid arthritis, White British)*

James also suggests a domestic cat as a metaphor for rheumatoid arthritis, indicating the aggressiveness of the condition isn't always the most salient issue, but importantly a cat holds all the control. A cat is unpredictable in when it will be friendly, and can represent a loss of control over day-to-day life, with rheumatoid arthritis dictating which will be good and bad days:

> *[A]nd a cat because cats just are aloof you know nobody controls the cat they control you and that's um … […] Yeah, no see a cat is quite good it can be friendly when it wants to be but when it doesn't want to be you know you can talk to the tail as they say. (James, 47yrs, rheumatoid arthritis, White British)*

Michael took a different approach to interpreting the question, "*If your rheumatoid arthritis were an animal, what animal would it be?*", and paints a strong image of his perception of rheumatoid arthritis and the loss of power and control he has experienced. Michael had been diagnosed for 10 years at the point of the interview. He was still experiencing a lot of anger related to the condition and diagnosis process and was struggling with acceptance. He did not like the idea of comparing rheumatoid arthritis to an animal, as he saw the condition as more sinister than an animal following its instinct:

> *Well, comparing it to say to someone in the animal kingdom, which are natural creatures in their natural environment, doing their natural things, I am not sure that's a good analogy to be honest with you. Um, you know because an animal doesn't attack you for no reason … because you are normally threatening it you know. If it's people, that would be different. (Michael, 48yrs, rheumatoid arthritis, White British)*

I invited Michael to answer the question in any way he would like to. His response provides a vivid metaphor for the loss of power and control to the point of helplessness that he felt due to the unpredictable and aggressive nature of rheumatoid arthritis:

> *Someone like Hannibal Lecter [notorious fictional psychopath and cannibal* (Harris, 1981, 1988)*] … Um, it's going to attack you at your lowest point and um where it hurts and um with malice in their heart really. Whereas animals, you see, they don't do that they will just react instinctively, and you know if it is attacking you, you have got a chance of defending yourself and shooting it and removing it as a threat you know. But if you have got someone that's cleverer than you are and it's on your case it's stalking you um, no you are not looking at an animal which is just doing its own thing so no I'm sorry I am not sure I can think of any animal even the most venomous you know they are in their own element. As I say for me it's Hannibal Lecter as a person … there is only one creature that does things out of malice and nastiness and that's your fellow human being really, and that is what your arthritis is really, it's attacking, it's turning your defences against you, your vulnerable points, your weak points in a way that hurts and you know catches you at your most awkward and most vulnerable and that's what your psychiatrist turned serial killer does isn't it really that's their raison d'être really that's their theme*

Whilst the animal metaphors came from prompting participants to think about rheumatoid arthritis in this way, many of the other metaphors men used more naturally also captured this feeling of loss of power and control. John uses a metaphor of illness as a captor describing being constrained and trapped in a cage due to loss of mobility or movement:

> *The loss of mobility or the loss of freedom of movement I think, is, is extremely difficult to deal with when you're not used, when you're not accustomed to being constrained so it, it's extremely, again I find it extremely difficult and I've never experienced anything even remotely like it from that perspective. It's just, it's like you're in a cage, it's difficult. (John, systemic sclerosis, White British)*

Uncertainty and loss of control were also experienced in waiting for diagnosis and test results, which Arthur compares to the experience of taking school exams:

> *It's like having written an exam and waiting for your results ... you think you did okay but you don't know. (Arthur, late 60s, colon cancer, Canada)* (Wenger, 2013)

For some men, the loss of control of living with an uncertain future left them unable to see or focus on anything positive, using a commonly recognised metaphor of light representing hope:

> *I think that's one of the drawbacks that there's no light at the end of the tunnel, there's no cure. When you've got it, you can only think it's going to get worse, that's the worrying thing. (Brian, systemic sclerosis, White British)*

10.6 Barriers and Burdens

Men also used metaphors to describe the barriers and burdens experienced in daily life with a long-term condition. Loss of energy or strength was often compared to heavy immovable objects preventing them from going about their day. The impact of symptoms on daily life whether due to fatigue, pain, stiffness, or medication side effects were described as "*a lead weight*", "*walking into a brick wall*", and "*a bloody millstone*", representing their frustration with the restrictions living with a long-term condition can place on them.

James, who was unhappy at having had to give up playing rugby due to rheumatoid arthritis, included spiders in his response to the 'animal' question, with their webs representing the obstacles that long-term conditions can present to prevent him doing what he wanted to do:

> *You have got the spiders web because they're just continually thrown at you, you know spider and his web … its web is just continually being thrown out there … yeah you're there trying to fight your way through it and it keeps putting its web up to keep tracking you and stop you doing things that you want to do. (James, 47yrs, rheumatoid arthritis, White British)*

10.7 The Body as a Machine: Making Sense

Men seemed to use the metaphor of their body as a machine or piece of technology to explain or make sense of a long-term condition. Men with depression used these terms to indicate a cause outside of their control for their low mood, detaching themselves from the burden of responsibility: *"I'm made that way"*, *"My brain lacks the wiring for happiness"* (Clarke & Van Amerom, 2008), *"I am broken, I need to fix it but you know I can't exactly just go in with a screwdriver and just crack it open and duct tape it"* (Hoffman & Addis, 2021).

In an attempt to make sense of the cause of rheumatoid arthritis, Michael compares his body to a computer that has a virus. He extends this metaphor to go on to hypothesise an extreme cure:

> *It's almost like a computer virus, it's got an endless loop that won't stop. So, the question then is how do you solve that on a computer? Well, you can, well you pull the plug out and put it back in. So maybe with that analogy … the logical sort of follow-on from that maybe is um you know whether the body would redo that, you know, reboot its immune system, would it default back to the original factory setting? (Michael, 48yrs, rheumatoid arthritis, White British)*

The body as a machine metaphor has been seen previously in women with cancer (Gibbs & Franks, 2002). However, the example quotes provided for this metaphor in women (*"my body's working really hard for me"*, *"The disease broke me down"*, *"the doctor said we'd fix that"*) indicate a slightly different way this metaphor has been operationalised. These examples harness the metaphors of everyday language, whilst the men's technology-focused metaphors seem to be using a comparison between their body and their understanding of how technology and machinery work to provide insights into their condition. It is also possible that through using a metaphor of a machine, it helps men to dissociate or detach themselves from their body or mind, making it easier to cope with changes beyond their control.

10.8 Avoiding Crude Language

Finally, men would also turn to metaphors to avoid directly referring to sex, which may be due to embarrassment or discomfort in talking about this, or in some cases could be a way of lightening a topic that they may find difficult to discuss:

> *Well … it's like you're walking around with a loaded gun [functioning penis]. You feel more confident of yourself. (62yrs, moderate erectile dysfunction, Chinese)* (Low et al., 2009)

> *Yeah, you know, my wife says, you know, she may be available or whatever, she maybe a little bit amorous or whatever, you know, er, and you want to go and play football [have sex], you know, standing up, and you don't. (Paul, 52yrs, systemic sclerosis, White British)*

10.9 Summary

Men use a range of metaphors to discuss their experiences of living with a long-term condition, which seems to be a method of communication familiar to them. The metaphor most commonly picked up on in the literature for how men talk about a long-term condition is 'illness as war', with fighting and battle talk being commonly seen in men's discourses. However, this may be more of a product of common societal use of this metaphor in relation to illness and can also be found in women's narratives. Beyond the illness itself being discussed as an external force to be battled, men also talk about their bodies as playing both a hero and a villain role in their illness experience and in doing so split their bodies from the self as a separate entity to value or resent. Men's metaphors can indicate a way of coming to terms with altered masculine identities, describing lost 'superpowers' and using monstrous imagery to describe changes to appearance. Metaphors also depict the loss of power and control through the unpredictable and uncertain nature of living with a long-term condition, with the illness seen as a predator stalking, attacking, or capturing them. Men seem to use technology or mechanical metaphors to help make sense of and trouble-shoot their condition. Understanding the metaphors men use may be helpful in thinking about language used with men in clinic. Metaphors may be quite individual, and caution should be taken not to create misunderstanding through use of metaphors in place of direct language to convey clinically important information. However, listening and responding in kind to the metaphors men choose to use themselves could have the potential to support communication in clinic.

References

Arad, D. (2004). If your mother were an animal, what animal would she be? Creating play-stories in family therapy: The animal attribution story-telling technique (AASTT). *Family Process, 43*(2), 249–263.

Arroliga, A. C., Newman, S., Longworth, D. L., & Stoller, J. K. (2002). Metaphorical medicine: Using metaphors to enhance communication with patients who have pulmonary disease. *Annals of Internal Medicine, 137*(5 Part 1), 376.

Bettelheim, B. (2010). *The uses of enchantment: The meaning and importance of fairy tales* (3rd ed.). Vintage.

Bowker, J. (1996). Cancer, individual process, and control: A case study in metaphor analysis. *Health Communication, 8*(1), 91–104.

Cancer Research UK. (2023). *Cancer Research UK.* https://www.cancerresearchuk.org/

Clarke, J., & Van Amerom, G. (2008). A comparison of blogs by depressed men and women. *Issues in Mental Health Nursing, 29*(3), 243–264. https://doi.org/10.1080/01612840701869403

Clow, B. (2001). Who's afraid of Susan Sontag? Or, the myths and metaphors of cancer reconsidered. *Social History of Medicine, 14*(2), 293–312.

Connell, R. W., & Messerschmidt, J. W. (2005). Hegemonic masculinity rethinking the concept. *Gender & Society, 19*(6), 829–859.

Diabetes UK. (2023). *Diabetes UK.* https://www.diabetes.org.uk/

Gibbs, R. W., Jr., & Franks, H. (2002). Embodied metaphor in women's narratives about their experiences with cancer. *Health Communication, 14*(2), 139–165.

Harpham, W. S. (2010). View from the Other Side of the Stethoscope: Metaphor as Medicine. *Oncology Times, 32*(6), 16.

Harris, T. (1981). *Red Dragon.* Arrow Books.

Harris, T. (1988). *The silence of the lambs.* Arrow Books.

Hawkins, A. H. (1999). *Reconstructing illness: Studies in pathography* (Vol. 393, 2nd ed.). Purdue University Press.

Hoffman, E., & Addis, M. (2021). Dilemmas of agency and blame in men's talk about depression. *Psychology of Men & Masculinities, 22*(4), 669–677.

Klein, M. (1952). The origins of transference. In M. Klein (Ed.), *Envy and gratitude and other works 1946–1963* (pp. 48–57). Delacorte Press.

Lakoff, G., & Johnson, M. (1980). *Metaphors we live by* (Vol. 111). University of Chicago Press.

Low, W. Y., Ng, C. J., Choo, W. Y., & Tan, H. M. (2009). How do men perceive erectile dysfunction and its treatment? A qualitative study on opinions of men. *The Aging Male, 9*(3), 175–180. https://doi.org/10.1080/13685530600914601

Maersk, J., Larsen, J., Rosted, E., & Lindahl-Jacobsen, L. (2022). "When I can ride my bike, I think, am I at all as sick as they say?": An exploration of how men with advanced lung cancer form illness perceptions in everyday life. *European Journal of Cancer Care, 31*(6), e13751. https://doi.org/10.1111/ecc.13751

Mastergeorge, A. M. (1999). Revelations of family perceptions of diagnosis and disorder through metaphor. In *Constructing (in) competence: Disabling evaluations in clinical and social interaction*. Lawrence Erlbaum Associates.

McArthur, T. (1992). *The Oxford companion to the English language*. Oxford University Press.

Mitchell, G., Ferguson-Pare, M., & Richards, J. (2003). Exploring an alternative metaphor for nursing: Relinquishing military images and language. *Nursing Leadership (Toronto, Ont.), 16*(1), 48–58.

Modell, A. H. (2005). Emotional memory, metaphor, and meaning. *Psychoanalytic Inquiry, 25*(4), 555–568.

Otto, M. W. (2000). Stories and metaphors in cognitive-behavior therapy. *Cognitive and Behavioral Practice, 7*(2), 166–172.

Peterson, J. W., & Sterling, Y. M. (2009). Children's perceptions of asthma: African American children use metaphors to make sense of asthma. *Journal of Pediatric Health Care, 23*(2), 93–100.

Quaglia, V. (2020). Men, masculinities and diabetes: 'Doing gender' in Italian men's narratives of chronic illness. *Sociology of Health & Illness, 42*(8), 1902–1917. https://doi.org/10.1111/1467-9566.13176

Quincey, K., Williamson, I., & Winstanley, S. (2016). 'Marginalised malignancies': A qualitative synthesis of men's accounts of living with breast cancer. *Social Science & Medicine, 149*, 17–25. https://doi.org/10.1016/J.SOCSCIMED.2015.11.032

Reisfield, G. M., & Wilson, G. R. (2004). Use of metaphor in the discourse on cancer. *Journal of Clinical Oncology, 22*(19), 4024–4027.

Richardson, J., & Grose, J. (2009). The use of descriptive words and metaphor in patient and carer experience of palliative day care: Secondary analysis of a qualitative study. *The Open Nursing Journal, 3*, 18–24.
Snell, G. E., Seage, C. H., & Mercer, J. (2023). A phenomenological study on the lived experience of men with chronic fatigue syndrome. *Journal of Health Psychology*. https://doi.org/10.1177/13591053231186385
Stand up to cancer. (2023). *Stand up to cancer*. https://www.standuptocancer.org.uk/
Stapleton, S., & Pattison, N. (2014). The lived experience of men with advanced cancer in relation to their perceptions of masculinity: A qualitative phenomenological study. *Journal of Clinical Nursing, 24*(7–8), 1069–1078. https://doi.org/10.1111/jocn.12713
Wenger, L. (2013). "Living under assault": Men making sense of cancer. *European Journal of Cancer Care, 22*, 389–399. https://doi.org/10.1111/ecc.12042
Whaley, B. B. (2000). Explaining illness to children: Theory, strategies, and future inquiry. In B. B. Whaley (Ed.), *Explaining illness: Research, theory and strategies* (Vol. Issue 2, pp. 191–203). Lawrence Erlbaum Associates.
Wurmser, L. (2011). Metaphor as conflict, conflict as metaphor. *Psychoanalytic Inquiry, 31*(2), 107–125. https://doi.org/10.1080/07351690.2010.515528

CHAPTER 11

Tips for Supporting Men

Drawing together the evidence and discussion that I've presented throughout this book I'll leave you with three groups of 'top ten tips' for healthcare professionals, researchers, and anyone looking to create support services for men with long-term conditions to support you in taking a gender-sensitised approach. I'm not the first (and I certainly won't be the last!) to create suggestions for supporting and engaging men in relation to health. Similar ideas and suggestions can also be found in recent publications: the 5C Framework (Galdas et al., 2023) and eight lessons learnt from community-based men's health promotion programmes (Oliffe et al., 2020), both of which I drew on in writing Chap. 9.

11.1 Ten Tips for Healthcare Professionals Working with Men with Long-Term Conditions

If you're a busy healthcare professional who wants to know how you can better take a gender-sensitised approach to supporting men in your day-to-day clinics, this is for you. Here are my top ten tips for engaging and supporting men with long-term conditions:

1. **Address mental wellbeing**
   Whether you work in primary, secondary, or tertiary care, you have limited time per patient and a lot to get through. What if you ask about mental health or wellbeing and open a can of

C. Flurey, *Talking Men's Health*,
https://doi.org/10.1007/978-3-031-62593-0_11

worms you can't close and there's no time left for talking about the physical symptoms? As I've discussed throughout this book, mental and physical health are so interlinked it's hard to effectively treat one without addressing the other.

Men tend to assume that your focus is their physical health, so if you are asking about their mental wellbeing try to be explicit in this and avoid general questions like "How are you doing today?", which tend to be interpreted in relation to their physical symptoms. In clinical practice, you'll be used to visual analogue scales and numerical rating scales, so why not add in one more. Men can find it easier to start with a number rather than words in thinking about their feelings, so I'd recommend asking men about their 'mental fitness' using Talk Club's "How are you? Out of 10?". Then ask why this number (especially if it's low).

With limited time in clinic and a postcode lottery on psychological support services, social prescribing can be a useful tool. Is there a local Talk Club (Talk Club, 2024), Andy's Man Club (Andy's Man Club, 2022), Men's Sheds (Men's Sheds, 2024), or other male-focused group in your area? It is worth noting these groups are not always equipped to deal with serious mental health concerns, so for men repeatedly scoring in the lower end of the scale (the scale is not validated for a cut-off point) referral to formal psychological support should still be pursued.

2. **Ask about sex**

Sex and intimacy are important to men in achieving and maintaining their quality of life, but they can find this embarrassing to raise with you. I know it can sometimes feel awkward for you too, but they want you to ask—and if they don't have any issues to talk about they don't mind you asking—so what have you got to lose!

If you are concerned about a potentially awkward interaction, one solution is to provide patients with a sheet of paper with key words (e.g., sex and intimacy, medication, pain, etc.) and ask them to circle the things they would like to talk about while they are waiting for their appointment. The inclusion of sex and intimacy then highlights this is a topic you also consider important and is available for discussion.

For conditions that have the potential to cause erectile dysfunction, it's important to tell men this at diagnosis. In complex conditions you may understandably be wary of reeling off a list of potential symptoms at diagnosis. However, it can be particularly important to highlight erectile dysfunction to ensure men feel comfortable to tell you about this. As discussed in Chap. 5, the impact on sex and intimacy goes beyond erectile dysfunction so should be considered as a potential topic for discussion for men with all long-term conditions.

3. **Provide information**
   Men have been described as 'hungry for information' (Galdas et al., 2014); they tend to want to become experts in their condition. As with all patients there will be individual differences between men in when and how they would like to receive information. Men seemed to value clinicians who gave them information that was pitched at the right level for them, which will come from getting to know your patients over time. Be aware that while some men may be satisfied with patient information leaflets and signposting to charity websites, others would value being signposted towards academic papers. Men are likely to seek out information at their own pace so providing suggestions of helpful sources may avoid them discovering misinformation. It may also be helpful to ask men what they have learnt through their own research about their condition to enable misinformation to be corrected. This will also provide insight into their level of understanding and interest to tailor information provision.
   It is also useful to bear in mind that some men may rely on their partners to gather information, so involving them in the information-giving processes can be helpful. However, be cautious of pitching information at a partner's level of health literacy over the man's. Additionally, be aware that unpartnered men may need additional informational support. Check men's understanding of what you tell them to enable them to actively participate in their own health and self-management. If in doubt, one way of doing this is asking them to explain to you what you've told them.
4. **Don't be afraid to use humour**
   Men often use humour to discuss difficult topics and value when healthcare professionals match their humour. Whilst this may be harder with newly diagnosed patients, over time men with long-term conditions value healthcare professionals who get to know their humour and use it to lighten consultations. As I discussed in Chap. 6, dark humour (or gallows humour) can often be protective and help men to open up about fears they may not feel comfortable to directly voice. Being aware of this use of humour

can help to listen to what men may be indirectly telling you about their worries. However, dark humour may be best reserved for patients who you have got to know better as it can sometimes be unwelcome without (indirect) permission.

5. **Talk to men about death**
This advice won't apply to all long-term conditions, but if you're treating men with a life-limiting condition don't shy away from the subject. Men would like to talk about the emotional as well as medical side of death, but won't necessarily bring this up themselves. Men were interested in understanding more about the process of dying—would it hurt, what would it feel like. Men may not want to talk about death in front of their loved ones as they attempt to protect them, so do give them the opportunity to talk about this away from others. Provide multiple opportunities to discuss this topic, as they may not be ready the first time you ask. Finally, remember the powerful quote in Chap. 6: "*It's difficult to talk about your death to someone who may not be that interested in your life*" (Abbott et al., 2017). To talk meaningfully to men about death, first get to know who they are in life.
6. **Involve partners (but enable one-to-one consultations)**
Men in relationships tend to cope as a team with their partners. They often attend clinical appointments with their partners, and partner or family influence can encourage help-seeking behaviours. Involving partners in discussions can be an effective way of supporting self-management. Men can be encouraged or discouraged from engaging in health behaviours based on the attitudes and support of their partners, so getting them on board can be a crucial step in supporting self-management. However, it is important to note that some men feel a sense of responsibility to protect their partners from the full impact of their condition. This means if partners are present in all consultations, then men may find it difficult to open up about things that are worrying them. Men may not always find it easy to ask partners to step out of the room. Thus, it could be helpful to ask partners to leave for the first or last few minutes of a consultation to enable you to ask men about anything they would like to discuss. This may involve directly asking about issues mentioned above such as mental wellbeing, sex and intimacy, or mortality. Also remember not all men are partnered or have family support. It may be particularly

important to consider signposting these men to support services (e.g., those mentioned in point 1).

7. **Support men to stay in work**
   For many men, remaining in paid work is important to their sense of masculinity and psychological wellbeing. Where possible, support men to remain in employment. This could be through discussing ways to fulfil their work role through adjustments and work-arounds, relinquishing certain tasks, or considering changes of roles. This could also include providing information for men to share with their employers to support them in the workplace. It is often harder to return to work than to remain in work on light duties. Of course I'm not suggesting putting pressure on men to remain in a role that causes them more harm than good. However, a number of men discussed having to 'convince' their doctors they were well enough to keep working. So, where possible work with men to find a way to keep them working safely for as long as possible within the limits of their condition.
8. **Gamify self-management**
   In encouraging men to make lifestyle changes to manage a long-term condition, you might consider trying 'gamifying' it. This means turning self-management into a game or competition (against either themselves or others)—with achievable goals. For example, step counts could be used to increase movement with challenges to improve previous targets. Sharing men's biomarkers with explanation can also be a powerful tool in making them an active participant in their healthcare and setting targets to reduce or increase their 'numbers' (as applicable) through suggested behaviour changes.
9. **Reduce power imbalances**
   Being diagnosed with a long-term condition can cause men to feel a loss of power and control in their lives. They discussed valuing healthcare professionals who made an effort to reduce the power imbalance in medical consultations. This could be achieved in a variety of ways, such as using lay language and taking time to ensure patients understand procedures, tests, and investigations. It can also be through listening to patients and acknowledging the expertise they bring to the consultation as someone living with the condition.

10. **Be mindful of differences**
    Men are of course not an homogeneous group and will have different needs and preferences depending on their social, cultural, and individual differences. However, throughout the literature men discuss issues of conscious and unconscious biases affecting their experiences of and access to healthcare. If you're reading this section, I am probably preaching to the converted, but it bears repeating. Be cautious of approaching all consultations through a straight, white, middle-class lens. Small changes such as not making an assumption that a partnered man has a female partner can make a big difference in a patient feeling able to trust you to handle their specific concerns sensitively.

11.2 Ten Tips for Researchers Working with Men with Long-Term Conditions

It's so important to include men in health research to ensure that resulting outputs such as healthcare services or patient-reported outcome measures reflect the needs and experiences of men and women equally. I'm often approached by clinical researchers who are looking to increase the number of male participants in their studies. Even in mixed gender studies, if you're looking for equal numbers it's important to think about men from the start and develop recruitment materials that appeal to them. Here are ten tips from me for how to recruit and engage men in research studies:

1. **Study recruitment: Tell men you're looking for men**
   Whether your study focuses solely on men or whether you're looking for more of a gender balance in your mixed gender study the first piece of advice I will always give is if you're looking for men then tell them. Take the time to create research materials that specifically call out to men from the top of the page. Tell them why you need to hear from men without blaming them. For example, "Previous research has focused on more women than men and we don't know if men have a different experience". I'd avoid saying "no men have taken part so far" as this may make them feel less like 'normal' men if they do take part. Instead, focus on why it's important you hear from men. Throughout this book I've mentioned how men like to become experts in their condition. Telling them you need this expertise can be powerful.

2. **Study recruitment: Think about who your gatekeepers are**
   It can be important to men that the use of their time in the study you're trying to recruit them to is well spent. One measure of this is that people whose opinion they value have validated the study as worthwhile. Thus, whilst gatekeepers can sometimes create additional barriers to study recruitment, they can also be used to provide legitimacy. For men with long-term conditions this is likely to be a member of their clinical team. However, it could also be trusted members of their community, or facilitators of charity groups that they are part of (e.g., patient charities). Additionally, men's spouses or partners can also act as gatekeepers; they may hold the social calendar for both of them and can be valuable in encouraging men to take part.
3. **Study recruitment: Be clear about the purpose**
   Be clear about the purpose of the research study, what it will involve, and how long it will take. Men value taking part in things that have a clear purpose so make sure you tell them why you're doing this and what difference they can make. Whilst drug trials offer a clear potential benefit, it can sometimes be harder to see the clinical value of a qualitative study or psychosocial study. So, it's important to explain this, but do be careful not to over-promise or over-exaggerate the difference your study can make. It may mean explaining additional research studies that will be needed to follow on from this that your study will feed into.
4. **Gender-sensitise the language of recruitment material**
   In Chap. 9 I discussed the power of gender-sensitising interventions for men in both language and style, and this is also relevant for recruiting men to research studies. Think about the language you're using in your participant information sheets, whilst still being honest about what the study focus will be. For example, "We'd like to understand what we could do to improve your care" may be better received than "We'd like to understand your support needs". 'Mental fitness' may be more acceptable than 'mental health'. Emphasising the need to learn from men's expertise in the condition can also add value. If you're highlighting a lack of previous research with men, try and frame this according to a lack of researcher's ability to previously engage men in research, rather than using blaming language that implies a lack of previous engagement from men.

5. **Allow time to talk about safe topics and give permission to open up**
   In both focus groups and interviews start with broad questions that enable men to interpret it in a way that allows them to discuss 'safe topics' (e.g., symptoms, medication, side effects). Build rapport and trust first through these before moving on to topics that require more vulnerability, such as focusing on emotional impact. This can be particularly important in focus groups as men need time to build rapport with and 'position' themselves against the other men in the group. Remember that for many men, this may be the first time they've spoken to another man with the same condition. They've given you their time to provide you with data, so allow them the time to develop their knowledge by comparing symptoms and medication with each other. For topics that may be trickier because they may be emotive or embarrassing, give men permission to talk about these by addressing them directly. Men often want to talk about these issues but may need reassurance you're expecting to hear them.
6. **Be flexible**
   Try and be as flexible as possible. This can mean offering a combination of interviews and focus groups to provide options that appeal to men's preferences or availability. It might also mean being flexible on the length of time you were anticipating an interview might take. For example, I've had men give me 45 minutes in their lunch break and I've been selective in the parts of the interview schedule I focused on, which was preferable to losing the interview completely. I've also run focus groups in the evening to catch men who added the study on to the end of the working day. If possible, also offer both online and in-person options for data collection. For interviews, I've also provided the option of interviewing men in their homes. This was rarely taken up by men unless they had mobility issues, which may reflect the dynamic of me being a female researcher.
7. **Consider the gender split in focus groups**
   Men had differing views on whether they preferred support to be male-only or mixed-gender groups. However, many men said they would not have talked about certain topics (e.g., erectile dysfunction) or talked so openly if female patients had been present. Additionally, whilst some men didn't mind mixed-gender groups, they were sometimes put off being the only man in a group or

being noticeably outnumbered. Thus, if you're planning a mixed gender study with groups, I would advise looking at your gender split. Depending on the topic it may not be necessary or appropriate to split by gender, but if focusing on illness experiences this may be worth considering. Nevertheless, it would be advisable for men to not be noticeably outnumbered to avoid putting them off taking part in future.

8. **Don't worry so much about who you are**
   Does it matter that you're a woman or a man researching men? Which is better? Well, as with clinicians there's no real agreement in the literature or between men on whether they would prefer to speak to a male or female researcher. Of course, you may get a different narrative depending on who you are (including your other characteristics beyond your gender) but none of these are any more or less authentic. The important thing is providing a safe, private, and trusted space for men to open up. I found part of this trust included allowing men to ask me things about myself and being open with my responses.
9. **Men are not an homogeneous group**
   Finally, men are not an homogeneous group and it's important to remember that barriers to taking part in research exist that go beyond being a man. Throughout the book I discuss various ways that men may develop a lack of distrust in medicine or their healthcare professionals due to both explicit and implicit bias (e.g., towards ethnicity or sexuality). It is inevitable that this mistrust would carry through to health research, and much bridge building is needed between researchers and under-served communities to mend these gaps. Including representatives from the communities you are looking to research as equal partners in the research process is a good starting point to address this.
10. **Share your findings with participants**
    As I've highlighted throughout, men were often keen to learn more about their condition in many ways. One way of helping with this as a researcher is to share our findings with our participants. It's good practice whoever your participants are to share a lay summary of your findings. I would also suggest offering the option to receive a copy of the published paper in addition to the lay summary, as participants have varying levels of detail they would value. This also ensures that men see the finished product and the purpose of what they've given their time for, which may encourage future research participation.

11.3 Ten Tips for Designing Support Services/Interventions for Men with Long-Term Conditions

Finally, drawing together everything I've learnt from my own research and the literature, here are my top ten tips for developing support services or interventions for men with long-term conditions:

1. **Provide a clear shared purpose**
   Men want support to have a clear shared purpose. Mental wellbeing doesn't need to be the focus for there to be a psychological benefit to support. This shared purpose could be condition-specific such as an information giving session (see point 3), or a shared sport or physical activity to benefit self-management. It could include practical shared tasks such as the Men's Sheds model or even making pies together (like Men's pie club). In these activities, talking and providing support doesn't need to be the focus; they will occur naturally as a by-product of engaging together in shared activities. As I suggested in Chap. 9, creating a Men's Sheds space for men with long-term conditions to problem solve and create adaptive tools and devices together could be worth considering. The shared purpose of the group could also be talking itself—as exemplified by Talk Club. However, this still has a clear structure and the shared purpose of 'improving mental fitness'.
2. **Provide opportunity to talk**
   Whilst talking doesn't need to be the purpose or focus of a support intervention, provide the opportunity for it to happen. Leave space for men to talk through not packing every element with a facilitator or guest speaker talking. Build in lengthy coffee breaks to sessions that focus more on information giving. Provide space and opportunity to talk without forcing it. It can help to embrace silence to allow time for thought and self-reflection. For activity-based support, allow men time to focus on the activity-based content and for discussion to be focussed around that to enable bonds and rapport to develop rather than forcing topics of conversation. For talking groups, the opportunity to talk is right there, but direct questions about emotions, venting, or feelings can be helpful to give men permission to talk about these.

3. **Provide a way to learn**
   Men want to become experts in their condition. Including a way for them to learn more should be an important component of support. Men varied in the way they would like to receive information. Some were keen to hear about the most recent developments or current research in their condition, which could take the form of didactic information giving with an opportunity to ask questions. Others were interested in question-and-answer sessions with their medical consultant or a variety of healthcare professionals—this format enabled them to also learn from questions that other patients may ask that they hadn't thought about. Men also liked being able to learn from other patients' experiences and to be able to share their own expertise with others. This could be learning from people who were further along in their disease duration, or to share tips on self-management or adaptations. Including the men themselves in information sessions, as experts by lived experience, can help to reduce the power imbalance of researchers or clinicians holding all the knowledge.
4. **Consider the marketing**
   Often getting men into support interventions is the difficult part; once they have chosen one and committed, they will often stay. The way interventions for men are marketed can have a big impact on whether men engage with them or not in the first place. Consider using gendered language in naming services and the language used around it. Talk Club describing itself as a 'male mental fitness movement' with invitations to 'get mentally strong' and sessions led by 'coaches' not 'facilitators' are effective examples of this masculinised language. Keep information simple and be clear about what will happen (relating back to point 1 of support needing a clear purpose), and how long it will last. However, avoid perpetuating negative male stereotypes with language such as 'man up'. Consider where may be most effective to advertise your group to capture men who may be most in need of the services. For example, Football Fans in Training recruited male participants during football matches at football clubs, which even included announcements over the loudspeakers at half time.
5. **Be flexible**
   Often, self-management or support interventions can take the format of attendance every week for a certain number of weeks, per-

haps with a consolidation session a few weeks later. For research studies this regular attendance over a fixed period of time can be important for measuring the effectiveness of an intervention. However, in my survey study with men with rheumatoid arthritis they preferred a more flexible approach to attending support. I'd therefore suggest an approach that enables men to access according to their need and availability. For information sessions, this could mean an advertised timetable of content, enabling them to access according to their availability and interest. Ongoing rolling sessions enable men to build up a cohort of peers over time, which may in itself encourage regular attendance through connectedness and commitment to peers. Barriers to attending support can also be practical issues such as parking, distance to travel (especially for rare conditions), and fitting it in around work commitments. Thus, taking a flexible approach may also mean offering online options.

6. **Provide ways for men to progress**
   For some men, the opportunity to use their expertise to help others can be a motivator for attending support sessions. Initiatives that enable men to progress into leadership roles can be a way of maintaining their involvement. Once men reach a point where they may no longer see the need for support, a leadership or facilitation role can provide them with a purpose, which can also boost their self-esteem. For example, training men to become facilitators of an intervention they were previously a member of. Additionally, taking part in the training itself has the potential to provide covert support through the shared purpose with other men at the similar stage of wanting to give back to others.
7. **Involve partners or carers (but not every session)**
   Men in relationships often cope together with their partners, and throughout my own qualitative research and the literature they suggest including their partners in support interventions. This was in recognition of partners needing support for the impact on them; due to a desire for partners to better understand men's experiences of the condition; and due to partners taking an active role in supporting self-management of the condition. Thus, there is a good argument for involving partners in support interventions, particularly those that involve information giving or sharing.

However, it is important to note that not all men welcomed partner involvement in support interventions. For some men there are certain elements of support that they don't want to talk about in front of family members as they felt an urge to protect them. For unpartnered men they may feel ostracised and less able to open up amongst other men's partners. Some gay men have expressed feeling uncomfortable to talk candidly about sexual issues in the presence of female partners.

Thus, it may be worth considering a model of support where partners are invited intermittently (e.g., once a month for weekly sessions)—and this is made clear to all when this will be happening to enable men to opt out of these sessions. The format of man-to-man and side-by-side could be considered for 'partners' days' with men and their partners attending together for the first half and then splitting into two groups for the second half of each session.

8. **Consider the setting**
   Strong evidence suggests that meeting men where they are at, in spaces where they reside and frequent, can be effective in promoting health engagement such as screening and vaccination uptake. However, for long-term conditions men's treating hospital often becomes a place that they frequent for appointments. Thus, the familiarity of their treating hospital can make it an attractive location for receiving support. The hospital setting can also enable men with long-term conditions to 'box off' their condition from their everyday life. The effectiveness and preference for the setting may be dependent on the level of engagement with health services demanded of their condition. Thus, I don't have an answer of the 'right' place for a support intervention to be placed, just an encouragement to consider where might be right for your particular group (see also point 10).
9. **Be inclusive of men from marginalised groups**
   Men value sharing support with people similar to them to provide a sense of connectedness. Whilst for many men having the same condition provided sufficient similarity, those from marginalised groups sometimes felt like an 'outsider' and reported a sense of not belonging. For these men, having a condition in common is insufficient in spaces that don't make an effort to be inclusive of differences (e.g., sexuality, ethnicity). For men from marginalised groups having shared identities or social and cultural experiences

can be more important than the shared specific condition. Thus, a group specifically for gay men with long-term conditions, for example, may be preferred to a group for any men with a specific condition. However, in the absence of these, every effort should be made for groups to be as inclusive as possible (see point 10).

10. **Work with men to design services**

    It's becoming increasingly recognised that quality care comes from working with the people it is being designed for, to ensure it meets their needs. This is also known as co-production, in which services are designed, developed, tested, and implemented in partnership with the very people it is intended to serve. This is equally relevant to men's health services as any other health service provision. In fact, with health services critiqued for being too feminised it may be even more important to work with men to ensure any support services developed are acceptable and appealing to them. However, a note of caution on involving those who are easy to recruit to support the design of services. Those men who are sufficiently activated in their healthcare to be involved in service design may have different support needs or barriers to engaging in support than those who are harder to engage. Including men from marginalised groups in developing support can be a step towards ensuring their needs are met in resulting groups or interventions.

    In addition to working with men in developing support services within healthcare it is also important to involve healthcare professionals and commissioners. This helps ensure that any support developed will be feasible to implement in practice and sufficiently cost-effective to receive ongoing support.

11.4 Summary

This chapter has rounded off this book with three sets of top ten tips: for healthcare professionals, researchers, and anyone looking to create support services for men with long-term conditions. Healthcare professionals should ask men about mental wellbeing, sex, and death (as appropriate) as they value being given permission to talk about these. Men value healthcare professionals who give them information, understand their humour, and make an effort to reduce the power imbalance in a medical consultation. Researchers need to consider men from the recruitment stage of studies. Recruitment materials should consider gender-sensitised language, make it clear to men they are needed, and emphasise a clear purpose to the study. Gatekeepers (e.g., healthcare professionals) may be helpful in legitimising a study's purpose. For a qualitative study, allow time for men to discuss 'safe' topics before moving on to emotive issues, be as flexible as possible around practical arrangements, and consider the gender split in focus groups for mixed gender studies. Support provision for men should include a clear purpose, provide an opportunity to talk, and a way to learn about their condition. The setting also needs to be considered to provide a safe, trusted environment. Including men in designing support services can help to ensure their needs are met. Partners should be included in men's healthcare and support, but it is important to note this may sometimes inhibit emotional discussion from men. Men are not an homogeneous group, so interactions and support services need to be mindful of individual and cultural differences.

11.5 Conclusion

Throughout this book I have demonstrated that when given permission and provided with the right environment, men do talk about their health. They not only speak about the physical impact of health but will talk openly to researchers and each other about the emotional impact.

Long-term conditions can pose significant challenges to masculinity through limiting self-reliance, independence, and ways of enacting power and control. Men's self-worth and masculinity is often tied up in their occupational status and fulfilling protector and provider roles within the family. When these are challenged, men can question their purpose and value with associated impact on their mental wellbeing. Men are aware of social restrictions in emotional expression and may exert caution in who they will open up to and to what extent. Men's families can be an important source of support for mental wellbeing. However, some men can mask the full impact of their condition, feeling a responsibility to live up to a protector role, making it important that men have access to support beyond this.

In some conditions, men were impacted by visible differences, causing some to withdraw from social activities such as visiting fitness spaces to avoid exposing parts of their body. Men seemed to experience a particular impact on their masculine body image when their body reduced in size, and they lost muscle mass. Male 'banter' could be cruel with some experiencing negative comments about their visible differences, and some even experiencing discrimination due to their appearance. Sex and intimacy are highly valued by men in achieving positive quality of life, and challenges to this also challenges their masculinity. They would like healthcare professionals to ask about sex and intimacy as even though they are willing to talk, this can be embarrassing for them to raise themselves. For men with life-limiting long-term conditions, mortality is a constant background worry. They grieve the loss of their potential life, and living with an uncertain timeline challenges the ability to maintain control. They would like healthcare professionals to address the emotional as well as medical side of death and help to demystify the dying process.

Social narratives that men are poor at looking after their health, don't seek medical help, and don't take part in group support are unhelpful and inaccurate. The direct threat of a diagnosis of a long-term condition seemed to refocus men's attention on taking care of themselves. Men often found ways to work around any limitations and were keen to develop expertise in their condition. At times, men may use avoidance and apathy as coping strategies, which may need attention to ensure this doesn't lead to distress. Men don't seem to delay help-seeking any more than women do, but the reasons differ. Men may delay whilst assessing whether their symptoms are sufficiently serious to warrant attention. They may also worry about being seen by others as weak for seeking help unnecessarily or experience fear and embarrassment of the healthcare process or resulting outcomes such as diagnosis or surgery. Men may also be put off seeking help by previous negative experiences such as symptoms being dismissed, or direct or indirect discrimination, racism, or homophobia. Men may be encouraged to seek help by being prompted by a friend or family member, and the message that they will be taken seriously by healthcare services. Men do value peer support, where they can feel part of an 'insider' group to share experiences without having to explain themselves. Men will join groups, and they will open up when provided with a safe, private, trusted environment with the space to express themselves in language they feel comfortable with. Support services for men work best if they have a clear, shared purpose with emotional expression and support occurring as a by-product of this.

Whilst the body of research into men's health is constantly growing there are clear gaps in our understanding of the experiences of long-term conditions in men from marginalised groups. There is a lack of ethnic diversity throughout the long-term conditions literature, across conditions. There is also a lack of literature focusing on the experiences of gay or bisexual men, and papers that do exist primarily cover the impact on sex and intimacy often in relation to prostate cancer treatment. I could find no literature that specifically focused on trans-men's experiences of living with a long-term condition, although some exist on their access to and experiences of breast and cervical cancer screening, which was beyond the scope of this book. Finally, there are many long-term conditions where men's experiences are still to be explored, and these require attention to understand men's needs within the context of their specific condition.

Overall, I hope this book has given an insight into men's experiences of living with a long-term condition, and demonstrates that when given a safe environment and permission to talk, some men even surprised themselves with how easy they found it to open up:

> *It's amazing we've got three men here and a lady [CF—researcher], you know, and we're talking about it fairly well for round one! (Paul, 52yrs, systemic sclerosis, White British)*

References

Abbott, D., Prescott, H., Forbes, K., Fraser, J., & Majumdar, A. (2017). Men with Duchenne muscular dystrophy and end of life planning. *Neuromuscular Disorders, 27*(1), 38–44.

Andy's Man Club. (2022). *Andy's Man Club.* https://andysmanclub.co.uk/

Galdas, P., Darwin, Z., Kidd, L., Blickem, C., McPherson, K., Hunt, K., Bower, P., Gilbody, S., & Richardson, G. (2014). The accessibility and acceptability of self-management support interventions for men with long term conditions: A systematic review and meta-synthesis of qualitative studies. *BMC Public Health, 14*(1), 1230.

Galdas, P. M., Seidler, Z. E., & Oliffe, J. L. (2023). Designing men's health programs: The 5C Framework. *American Journal of Men's Health, 17*(4). https://doi.org/10.1177/15579883231186463

Men's Sheds. (2024). *Men's Sheds.* https://menssheds.org.uk/

Oliffe, J., Rossnagel, E., Bottorff, J., Chambers, S., Caperchione, C., & Rice, S. (2020). Community-based men's health promotion programs: Eight lessons learnt and their caveats. *Health Promotion International, 35*, 1230–1240.

Talk Club. (2024). *Talk Club.* https://talkclub.org/

Glossary of Long-Term Conditions[1]

Alopecia areata is a condition causing hair loss, often in small, round patches on the scalp or other body areas. The immune system mistakenly attacks hair follicles, leading to hair thinning or complete loss. The exact cause is unclear, but genetics and environmental factors may contribute. Alopecia areata can affect anyone, including children, and its prevalence is approximately 2% worldwide.

Ankylosing Spondylitis (AS) is a type of arthritis affecting the spine and large joints, causing pain and stiffness. The immune system mistakenly attacks the joints' ligaments and bones, leading to inflammation and fusion of the spine. Symptoms include back pain, especially in the morning, and reduced flexibility. While the exact cause is unknown, genetics play a role. AS commonly starts in early adulthood. Until recently AS was thought to affect more men than women, but it is more recently thought to affect men and women equally. Exercise and medication can help manage symptoms, but there is no cure.

Anxiety is a common mental health condition marked by excessive worry and fear. Symptoms include restlessness, rapid heartbeat, sweating, and difficulty concentrating. The exact cause is a complex interplay of genetic, environmental, and brain chemistry factors. Stressful life events can trigger or exacerbate anxiety. It affects people of all ages, with

[1] Brief descriptions of the long-term conditions included in this book in alphabetical order.

C. Flurey, *Talking Men's Health*,
https://doi.org/10.1007/978-3-031-62593-0

approximately one in three individuals experiencing anxiety at some point. Treatment often involves therapy, medication, or a combination.

Asthma is a chronic respiratory condition causing airway inflammation and narrowing, leading to breathing difficulties. Symptoms include wheezing, shortness of breath, coughing, and chest tightness. Triggers like allergens or irritants exacerbate symptoms. While the exact cause is not fully understood, genetic and environmental factors contribute. Asthma often starts in childhood, but people of all ages can develop it. Globally, over 300 million individuals have asthma. Treatment involves inhalers to manage symptoms and lifestyle adjustments.

Barth syndrome is a rare genetic disorder affecting mainly men. It causes muscle weakness, fatigue, and problems with the heart, immune system, and growth. Individuals with Barth syndrome may experience low levels of certain fats in their cells, impacting energy production. The disorder is caused by mutations in a specific gene and is inherited from the mother. Its prevalence is estimated to be around 1 in 300,000 to 400,000 births. While there is no cure, supportive treatments aim to manage symptoms, including medications and therapies.

Cancer (breast) is a widespread form of cancer affecting breast cells. Symptoms may include a lump in the breast, changes in size or shape, and pain. While the exact cause is unclear, genetic factors and hormonal influences play a role. It's most common in women, but men can also develop it. Treatment options include surgery, chemotherapy, and radiation therapy.

Cancer (colon) is a type of cancer that affects the large intestine. Symptoms include changes in bowel habits, blood in the stool, abdominal discomfort, and unintentional weight loss. The exact cause is unclear, but factors like age, genetics, diet, and lifestyle contribute. It's prevalent among both men and women, with risk increasing with age. Treatment options may involve surgery, radiation, or chemotherapy.

Cancer (head/neck) involves tumours in the oral cavity, throat, or nasal passages. Symptoms encompass persistent sore throat, difficulty swallowing, voice changes, or a lump. Main causes include tobacco use, excessive alcohol consumption, and certain viral infections. It's more common in older individuals, particularly men. Treatment options may involve surgery, radiation, or chemotherapy.

Cancer (lung) is a serious condition where abnormal cells in the lungs grow uncontrollably, often leading to symptoms like persistent cough, chest pain, and breathlessness. Smoking, including passive exposure, is the leading cause, but non-smokers can also develop it due to various factors like genetics and environmental exposures. It is one of the most common cancers globally, affecting both men and women. Treatment involves surgery, chemotherapy, and radiation therapy.

Cancer (oral) affects the mouth and throat, with symptoms like persistent mouth sores, difficulty swallowing, and changes in voice. Primary causes include tobacco use, heavy alcohol consumption, and the human papillomavirus (HPV) infection. Globally, oral cancer is among the top cancers, more common in older adults, especially men. Treatment options may involve surgery, radiation, or chemotherapy.

Cancer (oropharyngeal) affects the throat, tonsils, or base of the tongue, with symptoms like persistent sore throat, difficulty swallowing, or voice changes. Main causes involve tobacco use, excessive alcohol, and human papillomavirus (HPV) infection. It's more common in men, often diagnosed in late stages. Treatment options may involve surgery, radiation, or chemotherapy.

Cancer (penile) affects the penis, with symptoms like lumps, sores, or changes in skin colour. Primary causes include smoking and human papillomavirus (HPV) infection. It's a rare cancer, more common in older men. Treatment options may involve surgery, radiation, or chemotherapy.

Cancer (prostate) affects the small gland producing seminal fluid, with symptoms like frequent urination, difficulty starting or stopping, and blood in urine. The exact cause is unclear, but age, family history, and ethnicity contribute. It's one of the most common cancers in men, with higher risk in older individuals. Early stages often exhibit no symptoms, emphasizing the importance of regular screenings, like the prostate-specific antigen (PSA) test. Treatment options range from active surveillance to surgery or radiation.

Cardiovascular disease (CVD) involves conditions affecting the heart and blood vessels, such as heart attacks and strokes. Symptoms include chest pain, shortness of breath, and fatigue. A variety of factors contribute to CVD, including high blood pressure, high cholesterol, smoking, and diabetes. Lifestyle choices, like a healthy diet and regular exercise, play a significant role. CVD is a leading global cause of death, impacting both men and women.

Chronic fatigue syndrome (CFS) is a complex, long-term condition characterized by persistent fatigue not alleviated by rest. Symptoms include profound tiredness, poor concentration, and unrefreshing sleep. The exact cause is unknown, but viral infections, immune system issues, and stress may contribute. CFS can affect anyone, often striking in early adulthood and more prevalent in women. Diagnosis relies on ruling out other conditions. No specific treatment exists, but managing symptoms through rest, pacing activities, and psychological support helps.

Coronary heart disease (CHD) is a common heart condition where blood vessels supplying the heart muscle become narrowed, leading to reduced blood flow. Symptoms include chest pain (angina), shortness of breath, and fatigue. The main cause is the build-up of fatty deposits in the coronary arteries, often linked to lifestyle factors like unhealthy diet and lack of exercise. CHD is prevalent worldwide, particularly in older adults. Risk factors include smoking, high blood pressure, and diabetes. Lifestyle changes, medications, and medical procedures like stents or bypass surgery help manage CHD.

Crohn's disease is a chronic inflammatory bowel condition causing symptoms such as abdominal pain, diarrhoea, weight loss, and fatigue. Its exact cause is unclear, but a combination of genetic, environmental, and immune system factors is involved. It commonly affects young adults, and while it can occur anywhere in the digestive tract, it often impacts the small intestine and colon. Crohn's is characterized by periods of flare-ups and remission. Treatment includes medications to reduce inflammation and manage symptoms, along with dietary changes.

Depression is a mental health condition marked by persistent feelings of sadness, hopelessness, and a lack of interest or pleasure in activities. Symptoms include changes in sleep patterns, appetite, and concentration, along with fatigue and low energy. While the exact cause is complex and involves biological, psychological, and environmental factors, stressful life events and genetics play a role. Depression affects people of all ages and backgrounds, with millions worldwide experiencing it. Treatment often involves therapy, medications, or a combination.

Depression (bipolar) involves extreme mood swings between depressive lows and manic highs. Symptoms during depressive episodes include profound sadness, fatigue, and changes in sleep and appetite. The cause is complex, influenced by genetic and environmental factors, and its onset often occurs in late adolescence or early adulthood. Bipolar depression affects millions globally, impacting personal relationships and daily functioning. Treatment involves mood-stabilizing medications and therapy to manage symptoms and prevent manic episodes.

Diabetes Mellitus is a chronic condition where blood sugar levels are consistently high. Symptoms include excessive thirst, frequent urination, and fatigue. The main causes involve genetics, lifestyle, and insulin resistance. There are two main types: Type 1, often diagnosed in childhood, and Type 2, more common in adults. In Type 1, the body doesn't produce insulin, while in Type 2, the body can't use insulin effectively. Diabetes affects millions globally, requiring daily management through medication, lifestyle changes, and monitoring blood sugar levels.

Duchenne muscular dystrophy is a genetic disorder causing progressive muscle weakness. Symptoms often begin in early childhood and include difficulty walking, frequent falls, and weakened muscles. DMD is caused by a mutation in the dystrophin gene, affecting muscle structure. It primarily affects boys, with an estimated incidence of 1 in 3500 live male births. There is currently no cure for DMD, but supportive treatments can alleviate symptoms and improve quality of life.

Fibromyalgia is a chronic condition causing widespread pain, fatigue, and tenderness in muscles, ligaments, and tendons. Common symptoms include sleep disturbances, difficulty concentrating (often called 'fibro fog'), and heightened sensitivity to touch. While the exact cause is unclear, factors like genetics, infections, and physical or emotional trauma contribute. It predominantly affects women and often surfaces between ages 30 and 60. Diagnosis relies on symptom assessment, as no specific tests confirm fibromyalgia. Management involves a multidisciplinary approach, incorporating medications, exercise, and stress reduction.

Inflammatory arthritis is the umbrella term for a group of disorders causing joint inflammation, leading to pain, swelling, and stiffness. It includes conditions like rheumatoid arthritis, psoriatic arthritis, and ankylosing spondylitis.

Obesity is a condition characterized by excess body weight, often resulting from an imbalance between calorie intake and expenditure. Symptoms include increased fat accumulation and associated health issues like diabetes, heart disease, and joint problems. Causes involve a combination of genetic, environmental, and lifestyle factors, with poor diet and lack of physical activity playing significant roles. Obesity affects people globally, with rising prevalence rates. Prevention and management entail adopting a balanced diet, regular exercise, and behavioural changes.

Osteoarthritis is a common joint condition causing pain and stiffness. Symptoms include joint pain, swelling, and reduced flexibility, often affecting knees, hips, and hands. The primary cause is the wear and tear of joint cartilage over time, leading to friction between bones. Age, genetics, and joint injuries contribute to its development. Osteoarthritis is prevalent in older adults but can affect people of all ages. There's no cure, but treatment involves pain management, exercise, and lifestyle adjustments.

Osteoporosis is a bone condition characterized by weakened and fragile bones, increasing the risk of fractures. Symptoms may not appear until a fracture occurs, often in the hip, spine, or wrist. The main cause is the loss of bone density, typically associated with ageing, hormonal changes, and inadequate calcium intake. It predominantly affects postmenopausal women, but men can also develop osteoporosis. Prevention involves a balanced diet rich in calcium and vitamin D, weight-bearing exercises, and lifestyle adjustments.

Parkinson's Disease is a progressive neurological disorder with symptoms like tremors, stiffness, and difficulty with balance and coordination. Its cause is linked to the loss of dopamine-producing cells in the brain, impacting movement control. While the exact cause is unclear, a combination of genetic and environmental factors plays a role. It usually affects people over 60, but younger individuals can develop early onset Parkinson's. There's currently no cure, but medications and therapies help manage symptoms.

Psoriatic Arthritis (PsA) is a chronic autoimmune disorder that causes joint pain, swelling, and stiffness, often affecting fingers, toes, and lower back. It affects about one in four people who already have the skin condition psoriasis (patches of red, flaky skin which is covered with silvery-like patches). Some people may develop psoriatic arthritis before the psoriasis is even present. In rare cases people have psoriatic arthritis and never have any noticeable patches of psoriasis. The exact cause is unknown, but both genetic and environmental factors contribute. PsA can develop at any age and affects men and women. Its onset is often linked to psoriasis flare-ups.

Raynaud's phenomenon is a condition affecting blood flow to certain parts of the body, usually fingers and toes. It leads to reduced blood supply, causing colour changes (white to blue to red) and numbness or tingling in extremities, especially in response to cold or stress. The exact cause is unclear, but it involves exaggerated blood vessel responses.

Raynaud's is more common in women and often appears in young adults. While it can be uncomfortable, management involves keeping warm and stress reduction.

Rheumatoid Arthritis (RA) is a chronic autoimmune disorder characterized by inflammation of the joints, causing pain, stiffness, and swelling. The immune system mistakenly attacks the synovium (the lining of membranes surrounding joints) leading to joint damage and deformities. RA's exact cause remains unclear, but involves genetic and environmental factors. It affects more women than men (around 70% women), and onset typically occurs between ages 30 and 60. Symptoms include joint pain, morning stiffness, fatigue, and systemic complications. Early diagnosis and intervention are crucial to managing RA, often involving medications and lifestyle changes. The prevalence of RA varies globally, affecting approximately 1% of the world's population.

Systemic Sclerosis (SSc also known as Scleroderma) is a rare autoimmune disease affecting the skin and internal organs. Symptoms include skin thickening, joint pain, Raynaud's symptoms, and problems with internal organs like the heart, lungs, and digestive system. Its exact cause is unknown, but it involves the immune system mistakenly attacking healthy tissues. Systemic sclerosis is more common in women and typically appears between the ages of 30 and 50. While there is no cure, treatment focuses on managing symptoms and preventing complications.

REFERENCES

Abbott, D., Jepson, M., & Hastie, J. (2016). Men living with long-term conditions: Exploring gender and improving social care. *Health & Social Care in the Community, 24*(4), 420–427. https://doi.org/10.1111/hsc.12222

Abbott, D., Prescott, H., Forbes, K., Fraser, J., & Majumdar, A. (2017). Men with Duchenne muscular dystrophy and end of life planning. *Neuromuscular Disorders, 27*(1), 38–44.

Alexander, J. (2001). Depressed men: An exploratory study of close relationships. *Journal of Psychiatric and Mental Health Nursing, 8*(1), 67–75. https://doi.org/10.1111/j.1365-2850.2001.00354.x

Alexis, O., & Worsley, A. J. (2018). A meta-synthesis of qualitative studies exploring men's sense of masculinity post-prostate cancer treatment. *Cancer Nursing, 41*(4), 298–310. https://doi.org/10.1097/NCC.0000000000000509

Anderson, B., Marshall-Lucette, S., & Webb, P. (2013). African and Afro-Caribbean men's experiences of prostate cancer. *British Journal of Nursing, 22*(22), 1296–1307. https://doi.org/10.12968/BJON.2013.22.22.1296

Andy's Man Club. (2022). *Andy's Man Club.* https://andysmanclub.co.uk/

Arad, D. (2004). If your mother were an animal, what animal would she be? Creating play-stories in family therapy: The animal attribution story-telling technique (AASTT). *Family Process, 43*(2), 249–263.

Arrington, M. I., Grant, C. H., & Vanderford, M. L. (2006). Man to man and side by side, they cope with prostate cancer: Self-help and social support. *Journal of Psychosocial Oncology, 23*(4), 81–102.

Arroliga, A. C., Newman, S., Longworth, D. L., & Stoller, J. K. (2002). Metaphorical medicine: Using metaphors to enhance communication with

C. Flurey, *Talking Men's Health*,
https://doi.org/10.1007/978-3-031-62593-0

patients who have pulmonary disease. *Annals of Internal Medicine, 137*(5 Part 1), 376.

Aurita, N., & Huda, M. (2018). Hierarchy of masculinities in George R.R. Martin's A Game of Thrones. In *Proceedings of The1st International Conference on Recent Innovations*, 614–621.

Avrech Bar, M., Dao, T. T., DeBlock Vlodarchyk, L. R., & Backman, C. L. (2021). Fatherhood experiences of men with inflammatory arthritis: A preliminary grounded theory. *Arthritis Care & Research, 73*(6), 885–892. https://doi.org/10.1002/ACR.24189

Ayhan, C. H. B., Bilgin, H., Uluman, O. T., Sukut, O., Yilmaz, S., & Buzlu, S. (2020). A systematic review of the discrimination against sexual and gender minority in health care settings. *International Journal of Health Services, 50*(1), 44–61. https://doi.org/10.1177/0020731419885093

Bamidele, O., McGarvey, H., Lagan, B. M., Parahoo, K., Chinegwundoh, M. B. E., & F., & McCaughan, E. (2019). "Man in the driving seat": A grounded theory study of the psychosocial experiences of Black African and Black Caribbean men treated for prostate cancer and their partners. *Psycho-Oncology, 28*(8), 1712–1720. https://doi.org/10.1002/PON.5150

Bates, J. S., & Taylor, A. C. (2012). Grandfather involvement and aging men's mental health. *American Journal of Men's Health, 6*(3), 229–239. https://doi.org/10.1177/1557988311430249

Bauer, G. (2016). Gender roles, comparative advantages and the life course: The division of domestic labor in same-sex and different-sex couples. *European Journal of Population, 32*(1), 99–128. https://doi.org/10.1007/S10680-015-9363-Z

Bay, L. T., Graugaard, C., Nielsen, D. S., Möller, S., Ellingsen, T., & Giraldi, A. (2020). Sexual health and dysfunction in patients with rheumatoid arthritis: A cross-sectional single-center study. *Sexual Medicine, 8*(4), 615–630. https://doi.org/10.1016/J.ESXM.2020.07.004

Bergner, E. M., Cornish, E. K., Horne, K., & Griffith, D. M. (2018). A qualitative meta-synthesis examining the role of women in African American men's prostate cancer screening and treatment decision making. *Psycho-Oncology, 27*(3), 781–790. https://doi.org/10.1002/pon.4572

Bettelheim, B. (2010). *The uses of enchantment: The meaning and importance of fairy tales* (3rd ed.). Vintage.

Bowker, J. (1996). Cancer, individual process, and control: A case study in metaphor analysis. *Health Communication, 8*(1), 91–104.

Branney, P., Witty, K., Braybrook, D., Bullen, K., White, A., & Eardley, I. (2014). Masculinities, humour and care for penile cancer: A qualitative study. *The Journal of Advanced Nursing, 70*(9), 2051–2060. https://doi.org/10.1111/jan.12363

Braun, V., & Clarke, V. (2021). *Thematic analysis: A practical guide*. SAGE.

British Society for Rheumatology, & Health Quality Improvement Partnership. (2022). *The national early inflammatory arthritis audit (NAIAA)*.

Broom, A., & Cavenagh, J. (2010). Masculinity, moralities and being cared for: An exploration of experiences of living and dying in a hospice. *Social Science & Medicine, 71*(5), 869–876. https://doi.org/10.1016/J.SOCSCIMED.2010.05.026

Brownhill, S., Wilhelm, K., Barclay, L., & Schmied, V. (2005). 'Big build': Hidden depression in men. *Australian and New Zealand Journal of Psychiatry, 39*(10), 921–931.

Bruun, D. M., Krustrup, P., Hornstrup, T., Uth, J., Brasso, K., Rørth, M., Christensen, J. F., & Midtgaard, J. (2014). "All boys and men can play football": A qualitative investigation of recreational football in prostate cancer patients. *Scandinavian Journal of Medicine & Science in Sports, 24*(SUPPL.1), 113–121. https://doi.org/10.1111/sms.12193

Bullen, K., Edwards, S., Marke, V., & Matthews, S. (2010). Looking past the obvious: Experiences of altered masculinity in penile cancer. *Psycho-Oncology, 19*(9), 933–940. https://doi.org/10.1002/pon.1642

Bunn, C., Palmer, V., Chng, N. R., Andersen, E., Gray, C. M., & Hunt, … Wyke, S. (2023). How European Fans in Training (EuroFIT), a lifestyle change program for men delivered in football clubs, achieved its effect: A mixed methods process evaluation embedded in a randomised controlled trial. *BMC Public Health, 23*(1). https://doi.org/10.1186/S12889-023-15419-Y

Busby, D. R., Horwitz, A. G., Zheng, K., Eisenberg, D., Harper, G. W., Albucher, R. C., Roberts, L. W., Coryell, W., Pistorello, J., & King, C. A. (2020). Suicide risk among gender and sexual minority college students: The roles of victimization, discrimination, connectedness, and identity affirmation. *Journal of Psychiatric Research, 121*, 182–188. https://doi.org/10.1016/J.JPSYCHIRES.2019.11.013

Campbell, R. D., & Mowbray, O. (2016). The stigma of depression: Black American experiences. *Journal of Ethnic and Cultural Diversity in Social Work, 25*(4), 253–269. https://doi.org/10.1080/15313204.2016.1187101

Cancer Research UK. (2023). *Cancer Research UK*. https://www.cancerresearchuk.org/

Capistrant, B. D., Torres, B., Merengwa, E., West, W. G., Mitteldorf, D., & Rosser, B. R. S. (2016). Caregiving and social support for gay and bisexual men with prostate cancer. *Psycho-Oncology, 25*(11), 1329–1336. https://doi.org/10.1002/pon.4249

Carretero, M. T., Calderón-Larrañaga, A., Poblador-Plou, B., & Prados-Torres, A. (2014). Primary health care use from the perspective of gender and morbidity burden. *BMC Women's Health, 14*(1), 145.

Clarke, J., & Van Amerom, G. (2008). A comparison of blogs by depressed men and women. *Issues in Mental Health Nursing, 29*(3), 243–264. https://doi.org/10.1080/01612840701869403

Connell, R. W. (2005). *Masculinities* (2nd ed.). University of California Press.

Connell, R. W., & Messerschmidt, J. W. (2005). Hegemonic masculinity rethinking the concept. *Gender & Society, 19*(6), 829–859.

Cooper, S., Leon, N., Namadingo, H., Bobrow, K., & Farmer, A. J. (2018). "My wife's mistrust. That's the saddest part of being a diabetic": A qualitative study of sexual well-being in men with Type 2 diabetes in sub-Saharan Africa. *PLOS ONE, 13*(9), e0202413. https://doi.org/10.1371/JOURNAL.PONE.0202413

Courtenay, W. H. (2000). Constructions of masculinity and their influence on men's well-being: A theory of gender and health. *Social Science & Medicine, 50*(10), 1385–1401.

Cramer, H., Horwood, J., Payne, S., Araya, R., Lester, H., & Salisbury, C. (2014). Do depressed and anxious men do groups? What works and what are the barriers to help-seeking? *Primary Health Care Research & Development, 15*(3), 287–301.

Culph, J., Wilson, N., Cordier, R., & Stancliffe, R. (2015). Men's Sheds and the experience of depression in older Australian men. *Australian Occupational Therapy Journal, 62*(5), 306–315. https://doi.org/10.1111/1440-1630.12190

De Visser, R. O., & McDonnell, E. J. (2013). "Man points": Masculine capital and young men's health. *Health Psychology, 32*(1), 5–14. https://doi.org/10.1037/A0029045

del Mar García-Calvente, M., Hidalgo-Ruzzante, N., del Río-Lozano, M., Marcos-Marcos, J., Martínez-Morante, E., Maroto-Navarro, G., Mateo-Rodríguez, I., & Gil-García, E. (2012). Exhausted women, tough men: A qualitative study on gender differences in health, vulnerability and coping with illness in Spain. *Sociology of Health & Illness, 16.*

Department of Health. (2012). *Long-term conditions compendium of Information: 3rd edition.*

Diabetes UK. (2023). *Diabetes UK.* https://www.diabetes.org.uk/

Donnelly, T. T., Suwaidi, J. M., Al-Qahtani, A., Asaad, N., & Singh, R. (2019). Arab men and women's conceptualization of mental health and depression: A qualitative study from the Middle East. *Journal of Immigrant and Minority Health, 21*(5), 1102–1114. https://doi.org/10.1007/S10903-018-0809-3

Doran, D., Williamson, S., Wright, K., & Beaver, K. (2018). "It's not just about prostate cancer, it's about being a gay man": A qualitative study of gay men's experiences of healthcare provision in the UK. *European Journal of Cancer Care, 27*(6), e12923. https://doi.org/10.1111/ecc.12923

Dougados, M., Soubrier, M., Antunez, A., Balint, P., Balsa, A., Buch, M. H., et al. (2014). Prevalence of comorbidities in rheumatoid arthritis and evaluation of their monitoring: Results of an international, cross-sectional study (COMORA).

Annals of the Rheumatic Diseases, 73(1), 62–68. https://doi.org/10.1136/annrheumdis-2013-204223

Doveson, S., Holm, M., Axelsson, L., Fransson, P., & Wennman-Larsen, A. (2020). Facing life-prolonging treatment: The perspectives of men with advanced metastatic prostate cancer—An interview study. *European Journal of Oncology Nursing, 49*. https://doi.org/10.1016/j.ejon.2020.101859

Dubin, J. M., Aguiar, J. A., Lin, J. S., Greenberg, D. R., Keeter, M. K., Fantus, R. J., Pham, M. N., Hudnall, M. T., Bennett, N. E., Brannigan, R. E., & Halpern, J. A. (2022). The broad reach and inaccuracy of men's health information on social media: Analysis of TikTok and Instagram. *International Journal of Impotence Research*, 1–5. https://doi.org/10.1038/s41443-022-00645-6

Dyer, K., & das Nair, R. (2013). Why don't healthcare professionals talk about sex? A systematic review of recent qualitative studies conducted in the United Kingdom. *The Journal of Sexual Medicine, 10*(11), 2658–2670. https://doi.org/10.1111/J.1743-6109.2012.02856.X

Eccleston, C., Williams, A. C., & Stainton Rogers, W. (1997). Patients' and professionals' understandings of the causes of chronic pain: Blame, responsibility and identity protection. *Social Science & Medicine, 45*(5), 699–709.

Edwards, R., Eccleston, C., & Keogh, E. (2017). Observer influences on pain: An experimental series examining same-sex and opposite-sex friends, strangers, and romantic partners. *Pain, 158*(5), 846–855. https://doi.org/10.1097/J.PAIN.0000000000000840

Emslie, C., Ridge, D., Ziebland, S., & Hunt, K. (2006). Men's accounts of depression: Reconstructing or resisting hegemonic masculinity? *Social Science & Medicine, 62*(9), 2246–2257.

Emslie, C., Ridge, D., Ziebland, S., & Hunt, K. (2007). Exploring men's and women's experiences of depression and engagement with health professionals: More similarities than differences? A qualitative interview study. *BMC Family Practice, 8*(43). https://doi.org/10.1186/1471-2296-8-43

Equality Act, c. 15 (2010). https://www.legislation.gov.uk/ukpga/2010/15/contents

Ervik, B., & Asplund, K. (2012). Dealing with a troublesome body: A qualitative interview study of men's experiences living with prostate cancer treated with endocrine therapy. *European Journal of Oncology Nursing, 16*(2), 103–108. https://doi.org/10.1016/J.EJON.2011.04.005

Fifield, J., Reisine, S., Sheehan, T. J., & McQuillan, J. (1996). Gender, paid work, and symptoms of emotional distress in rheumatoid arthritis patients. *Arthritis and Rheumatism, 39*(3), 427–435.

Fine, M., Weis, L., Addelston, J., & Marusza, J. (1997). (In)secure times: Constructing white working-class masculinities in the late 20th century. *Gender & Society, 11*(1), 52–68.

Flurey, C., Hewlett, S., Rodham, K., White, A., Noddings, R., & Kirwan, J. (2016a). Men, rheumatoid arthritis, psychosocial impact and self-management: A narrative review. *Journal of Health Psychology, 21*(10), 2168–2182. https://doi.org/1359105315572452

Flurey, C., Hewlett, S., Rodham, K., White, A., Noddings, R., & Kirwan, J. (2016b). "You obviously just have to put on a brave face": A qualitative study of the experiences and coping styles of men with rheumatoid arthritis. *Arthritis Care & Research, 69*(3), 330–337.

Flurey, C., Hewlett, S., Rodham, K., White, A., Noddings, R., & Kirwan, J. R. (2016c). Identifying different typologies of experiences and coping strategies in men with rheumatoid arthritis: A Q-methodology study. *BMJ Open, 6*(10), e012051. https://doi.org/10.1136/bmjopen-2016-012051

Flurey, C., Hewlett, S., Rodham, K., White, A., Noddings, R., & Kirwan, J. R. (2018a). Coping strategies, psychological impact and support preferences of men with rheumatoid arthritis: A multicentre survey. *Arthritis Care & Research, 70*(6), 851–860.

Flurey, C., Morris, M., Pollock, J., Richards, P., Hughes, R., & Hewlett, S. (2014a). Fluctuating balances: A Q-methodology study of flare help-seeking behaviours and different experiences of daily life in Rheumatoid Arthritis. *BMC Musculoskeletal Disorders, 15*, 364.

Flurey, C., Morris, M., Richards, P., Hughes, R., & Hewlett, S. (2014b). "It's like a juggling act": Rheumatoid Arthritis patient perspectives on daily life and flare whilst on current treatment regimes. *Rheumatology, 53*(4), 696–703.

Flurey, C., Pauling, J. D., Saketkoo, L. A., Denton, C. P., Galdas, P., Khanna, D., Williams, A., & Hughes, M. (2022). 'I turned in my man card': A qualitative study of the experiences, coping styles and support needs of men with systemic sclerosis. *Rheumatology, 62*(6), 2160–2167. https://doi.org/10.1093/RHEUMATOLOGY/KEAC585

Flurey, C., White, A., Rodham, K., Kirwan, J., Noddings, R., & Hewlett, S. (2018b). 'Everyone assumes a man to be quite strong': Men, masculinity and rheumatoid arthritis: A case-study approach. *Sociology of Health & Illness, 40*(1), 115–129.

Fox, K. (2004). *The Kleenex® for men crying game report: A study of men and crying*. http://webmail.sirc.org/publik/crying_game.pdf

Freeman, A., Mergl, R., Kohls, E., Székely, A., Gusmao, R., Arensman, E., Koburger, N., Hegerl, U., & Rummel-Kluge, C. (2017). A cross-national study on gender differences in suicide intent. *BMC Psychiatry, 17*(1), 1–11. https://doi.org/10.1186/S12888-017-1398-8

Frosh, S., Phoenix, A., & Pattman, R. (2002). *Young Masculinities*. Palgrave Macmillan.

Galdas, P., Darwin, Z., Kidd, L., Blickem, C., McPherson, K., Hunt, K., Bower, P., Gilbody, S., & Richardson, G. (2014). The accessibility and acceptability of self-management support interventions for men with long term conditions: A systematic review and meta-synthesis of qualitative studies. *BMC Public Health, 14*(1), 1230.

Galdas, P., Fell, J., Bower, P., Kidd, L., Blickem, C., McPherson, K., Hunt, K., Gilbody, S., & Richardson, G. (2015). The effectiveness of self-management support interventions for men with long-term conditions: A systematic review and meta-analysis. *BMJ Open, 5*(e006620). https://doi.org/10.1136/bmjopen-2014-006620

Galdas, P. M., Seidler, Z. E., & Oliffe, J. L. (2023). Designing men's health programs: The 5C Framework. *American Journal of Men's Health, 17*(4). https://doi.org/10.1177/15579883231186463

Gentili, C., McClean, S., Hackshaw-McGeagh, L., Bahl, A., Persad, R., & Harcourt, D. (2019). Body image issues and attitudes towards exercise amongst men undergoing androgen deprivation therapy (ADT) following diagnosis of prostate cancer. *Psycho-Oncology, 28*(8), 1647–1653. https://doi.org/10.1002/pon.5134

Gerbild, H., Areskoug-Josefsson, K., Larsen, C. M., & Laursen, B. S. (2021). Acceptability of health professionals' address of sexuality and erectile dysfunction—A qualitative interview study with men in cardiac rehabilitation. *Sexual Medicine, 9*(3). https://doi.org/10.1016/J.ESXM.2021.100369

Getachew, S., Tesfaw, A., Kaba, M., Wienke, A., Taylor, L., Kantelhardt, E. J., & Addissie, A. (2020). Perceived barriers to early diagnosis of breast Cancer in south and southwestern Ethiopia: A qualitative study. *BMC Women's Health, 20*(1). https://doi.org/10.1186/S12905-020-00909-7

Gibbs, R. W., Jr., & Franks, H. (2002). Embodied metaphor in women's narratives about their experiences with cancer. *Health Communication, 14*(2), 139–165.

Gibson, G., & Kierans, C. (2017). Ageing, masculinity and Parkinson's disease: Embodied perspectives. *Sociology of Health & Illness, 39*(4), 532–546. https://doi.org/10.1111/1467-9566.12508

Goodwill, J., Taylor, R., & Watkins, D. (2019). Everyday discrimination, depressive symptoms, and suicide ideation among African American men. *Archives of Suicide Research, 25*(1), 74–93. https://doi.org/10.1080/13811118.2019.1660287

Gough, B., Robertson, S., & Luck, H. (2021). Engendered expressions of anxiety: Men's emotional communications with women and other men. *Frontiers in Sociology, 6*. https://doi.org/10.3389/FSOC.2021.697356

Gray, C. M., Wyke, S., Zhang, R., Anderson, A. S., Barry, S., Brennan, G., Briggs, A., Boyer, N., Bunn, C., Donnachie, C., Grieve, E., Kohli-Lynch, C., Lloyd, S., Mcconnachie, A., Mccowan, C., Mclean, A., Mutrie, N., & Hunt, K. (2018). Long-term weight loss following a randomised controlled trial of a weight management programme for men delivered through professional football clubs: The Football Fans in Training follow-up study. *Public Health Research, 6*(9). https://doi.org/10.3310/phr06090

Grogan, S., & Richards, H. (2002). Body image. *Men and Masculinities, 4*(3), 219–232.

Groven, K., Galdas, P., & Solbrække, K. (2015). Becoming a normal guy: Men making sense of long-term bodily changes following bariatric surgery. *International Journal of Qualitative Studies on Health and Well-Being, 10*(1). https://doi.org/10.3402/qhw.v10.29923

Hackshaw-Mcgeagh, L. E., Sutton, E., Persad, R., Aning, J., Bahl, A., Koupparis, A., Millett, C., Martin, R. M., & Lane, J. A. (2017). Acceptability of dietary and physical activity lifestyle modification for men following radiotherapy or radical prostatectomy for localised prostate cancer: A qualitative investigation. *BMC Urology, 17*(1), 1–11. https://doi.org/10.1186/S12894-017-0284-5

Hamed, S., Bradby, H., Ahlberg, B. M., & Thapar-Björkert, S. (2022). Racism in healthcare: A scoping review. *BMC Public Health, 22*(988). https://doi.org/10.1186/s12889-022-13122-y

Hankerson, S. H., Suite, D., & Bailey, R. K. (2015). Treatment disparities among African American men with depression: Implications for clinical practice. *Journal of Health Care for the Poor and Underserved, 26*(1), 21–34. https://doi.org/10.1353/hpu.2015.0012

Harpham, W. S. (2010). View from the Other Side of the Stethoscope: Metaphor as Medicine. *Oncology Times, 32*(6), 16.

Harris, T. (1981). *Red Dragon.* Arrow Books.

Harris, T. (1988). *The silence of the lambs.* Arrow Books.

Hawkins, A. H. (1999). *Reconstructing illness: Studies in pathography* (Vol. 393, 2nd ed.). Purdue University Press.

Hayashi, S., Sato, K., Oishi, F., Fukuda, H., Hayama, Y., & Ando, S. (2023). Care needs of Japanese men for sexual dysfunction associated with prostate cancer treatment. *Supportive Care in Cancer, 31*(7), 1–9. https://doi.org/10.1007/S00520-023-07837-W

Helland, Y., Garratt, A., Kjeken, I., Kvien, T., & Dagfinrud, H. (2013). Current practice and barriers to the management of sexual issues in rheumatology: Results of a survey of health professionals. *Scandinavian Journal of Rheumatology, 42*(1), 20–26. https://doi.org/10.3109/03009742.2012.709274

Hendricks, E., Jenkinson, E., Falconer, L., & Griffiths, C. (2023). How effective are psychosocial interventions at improving body image and reducing disordered eating in adult men? A systematic review. *Body Image, 47*(101612). https://doi.org/10.1016/j.bodyim.2023.08.004

Hilton, S., Hunt, K., Emslie, C., Salinas, M., & Ziebland, S. (2008). Have men been overlooked? A comparison of young men and women's experiences of chemotherapy-induced alopecia. *Psych-Oncology, 17*(6), 577–583. https://doi.org/10.1002/pon.1272

Hinton, L., Apesoa-Varano, E. C., Unützer, J., Dwight-Johnson, M., Park, M., & Barker, J. C. (2015). A descriptive qualitative study of the roles of family members in older men's depression treatment from the perspectives of older men and primary care providers. *International Journal of Geriatric Psychiatry, 30*(5), 514–522. https://doi.org/10.1002/gps.4175

Hoffman, E., & Addis, M. (2021). Dilemmas of agency and blame in men's talk about depression. *Psychology of Men & Masculinities, 22*(4), 669–677.

Hu, T. W., Cooke, M., & McCarthy, A. (2009). A qualitative study of the experience of oral cancer among Taiwanese men. *International Journal of Nursing Practice, 15*(4), 326–333. https://doi.org/10.1111/J.1440-172X.2009.01759.X

Hughes, M., Pauling, J. D., Armstrong-James, L., Denton, C. P., Galdas, P., & Flurey, C. (2020). Gender-related differences in systemic sclerosis. In *Autoimmunity Reviews* (Vol. 19, Issue 4, p. 102494). Elsevier B.V. https://doi.org/10.1016/j.autrev.2020.102494

Hunt, K., Adamson, J., Hewitt, C., & Nazareth, I. (2011). Do women consult more than men? A review of gender and consultation for back pain and headache. *Journal of Health Services Research and Policy, 16*(2), 108–117. https://doi.org/10.1258/JHSRP.2010.009131

Hunt, K., Wyke, S., Gray, C. M., Anderson, A. S., Brady, A., Bunn, C., Donnan, P. T., Fenwick, E., Grieve, E., & Leishman, J. (2014). A gender-sensitised weight loss and healthy living programme for overweight and obese men delivered by Scottish Premier League football clubs (FFIT): A pragmatic randomised controlled trial. *The Lancet, 383*(9924), 1211–1221.

Ireland, D. (2019, August 11). *"Don't confuse your medical degree with my life"—Patient.* LinkedIn. https://www.linkedin.com/pulse/dont-confuse-your-medical-degree-my-life-patient-dawn-m-ireland/

Isano, S., Yohannes, T., Igihozo, G., Ndatinya, G. I., & Wong, R. (2023). A qualitative study to explore the healthcare-seeking experiences of men who have sex with men (MSM) and transgender women (TGW) in Rwanda. *BMC Health Services Research, 23*(1), 291. https://doi.org/10.1186/S12913-023-09286-X

Jaspers, E., & Verbakel, E. (2013). The division of paid labor in same-sex couples in the Netherlands. *Sex Roles, 68*, 335–348. https://doi.org/10.1007/S11199-012-0235-2

Johnson, J. L., Oliffe, J. L., Kelly, M. T., Galdas, P., & Ogrodniczuk, J. S. (2012). Men's discourses of help-seeking in the context of depression. *Sociology of Health & Illness, 34*(3), 345–361. https://doi.org/10.1111/J.1467-9566.2011.01372.X

Jonsson, A., Aus, G., & Bertero, C. (2009). Men's experience of their life situation when diagnosed with advanced prostate cancer. *European Journal of Oncology Nursing, 13*, 268–273.

Jowett, A., Peel, E., & Shaw, R. L. (2011). Sex and diabetes: A thematic analysis of gay and bisexual men's accounts. *Journal of Health Psychology, 17*(3), 409–418. https://doi.org/10.1177/1359105311412838

Juel, K., & Christensen, K. (2008). Are men seeking medical advice too late? Contacts to general practitioners and hospital admissions in Denmark 2005. *Journal of Public Health, 30*(1), 111–113. https://doi.org/10.1093/pubmed/fdm087

Kazer, M. W., Harden, J., Burke, M., Sanda, M. G., Hardy, J., & Bailey, D. E. (2011). The experiences of unpartnered men with prostate cancer: A qualitative analysis. *Journal of Cancer Survivorship, 5*(2), 132–141. https://doi.org/10.1007/S11764-010-0157-3

Khazen, M. (2022). Power dynamics in doctor-patient relationships: A qualitative study examining how cultural and personal relationships facilitate medication requests in a minority with collectivist attributes. *Patient Education and Counselling, 105*(7), 2038–2044.

Klafke, N., Eliott, J., Olver, I., & Wittert, G. (2014). Australian men with cancer practice complementary therapies (CTs) as a coping strategy. *Psycho-Oncology, 23*(11), 1236–1242. https://doi.org/10.1002/pon.3550

Klein, M. (1952). The origins of transference. In M. Klein (Ed.), *Envy and gratitude and other works 1946–1963* (pp. 48–57). Delacorte Press.

Lack, S., Noddings, R., & Hewlett, S. (2011). Men's experiences of rheumatoid arthritis: An inductive thematic analysis. *Musculoskeletal Care, 9*(2), 102–112. https://doi.org/10.1002/msc.203

Lakoff, G., & Johnson, M. (1980). *Metaphors we live by* (Vol. 111). University of Chicago Press.

Lambert, S. D., & Loiselle, C. G. (2008). Combining individual interviews and focus groups to enhance data richness. *Journal of Advanced Nursing, 62*(2), 228–237.

Langelier, D. M., Jackson, C., Bridel, W., Grant, C., & Culos-Reed, S. N. (2022). Coping strategies in active and inactive men with prostate cancer: A qualitative study. *Journal of Cancer Survivorship, 16*(2), 421–431. https://doi.org/10.1007/S11764-021-01037-3

Latreille, S., Collyer, A., & Temple-Smith, M. (2014). Finding a segue into sex: Young men's views on discussing sexual health with a GP. *Australian Family Physician, 43*(4), 217–221.

Lee, S., Schorr, E., Hadidi, N. N., Kelley, R., Treat-Jacobson, D., & Lindquist, R. (2018). Power of peer support to change health behavior to reduce risks for heart disease and stroke for African American men in a faith-based community. *Journal of Racial and Ethnic Health Disparities, 5*(5), 1107–1116. https://doi.org/10.1007/S40615-018-0460-7

Letts, C., Tamlyn, K., & Byers, E. S. (2010). Exploring the impact of prostate cancer on men's sexual well-being. *Journal of Psychosocial Oncology, 28*(5), 490–510. https://doi.org/10.1080/07347332.2010.498457

Lim, S. S., Vos, T., Flaxman, A. D., Danaei, G., Shibuya, K., Adair-Rohani, H., AlMazroa, M. A., Amann, M., Anderson, H. R., & Andrews, K. G. (2012). A comparative risk assessment of burden of disease and injury attributable to 67 risk factors and risk factor clusters in 21 regions, 1990–2010: A systematic analysis for the Global Burden of Disease Study 2010. *The Lancet, 380*(9859), 2224–2260.

Lockwood Estrin, G., Milner, V., Spain, D., Happé, F., & Colvert, E. (2021). Barriers to Autism Spectrum Disorder diagnosis for young women and girls: A systematic review. *Review Journal of Autism and Developmental Disorders, 8*(4), 454–470. https://doi.org/10.1007/S40489-020-00225-8

Low, W. Y., Ng, C. J., Choo, W. Y., & Tan, H. M. (2009). How do men perceive erectile dysfunction and its treatment? A qualitative study on opinions of men. *The Aging Male, 9*(3), 175–180. https://doi.org/10.1080/13685530600914601

Maersk, J., Larsen, J., Rosted, E., & Lindahl-Jacobsen, L. (2022). "When I can ride my bike, I think, am I at all as sick as they say?": An exploration of how men with advanced lung cancer form illness perceptions in everyday life. *European Journal of Cancer Care, 31*(6), e13751. https://doi.org/10.1111/ecc.13751

Mannix, K. (2022, November). *What happens as we die?* TEDx.

Mastergeorge, A. M. (1999). Revelations of family perceptions of diagnosis and disorder through metaphor. In *Constructing (in) competence: Disabling evaluations in clinical and social interaction*. Lawrence Erlbaum Associates.

Matcham, F., Norton, S., Scott, D. L., Steer, S., & Hotopf, M. (2015). Symptoms of depression and anxiety predict treatment response and long-term physical health outcomes in rheumatoid arthritis: Secondary analysis of a randomized controlled trial. *Rheumatology, 55*(2), 268–278.

Matheson, L., Watson, E., Nayoan, J., Wagland, R., Glaser, A., Gavin, A., Wright, P., & Rivas, C. (2017). A qualitative metasynthesis exploring the impact of prostate cancer and its management on younger, unpartnered and gay men. *European Journal of Cancer Care, 26*(6). https://doi.org/10.1111/ecc.12676

Mazar, I., & Moorman, S. M. (2021). "I want that life a lot…how on earth do I get that?" Examining challenges for men with Barth Syndrome in their transitions to adulthood. *Journal of Patient Experience, 8*. https://doi.org/10.1177/23743735211060783

McArthur, T. (1992). *The Oxford companion to the English language*. Oxford University Press.

McCaughan, E., Prue, G., Parahoo, K., McIlfatrick, S., & McKenna, H. (2011). Exploring and comparing the experience and coping behaviour of men and women with colorectal cancer at diagnosis and during surgery. *Journal of Advanced Nursing, 67*(7), 1591–1600.

McConkey, R. W., & Holborn, C. (2018). Exploring the lived experience of gay men with prostate cancer: A phenomenological study. *European Journal of Oncology Nursing, 33*, 62–69. https://doi.org/10.1016/j.ejon.2018.01.013

McCormack, M., & Anderson, E. (2010). "It's just not acceptable any more": The erosion of homophobia and the softening of masculinity at an English sixth form. *Sociology, 44*(5), 843–859. https://doi.org/10.1177/0038038510375734

McDonagh, L. K., Nielsen, E. J., McDermott, D. T., Davies, N., & Morrison, T. G. (2017). "I want to feel like a full man": Conceptualizing gay, bisexual, and heterosexual men's sexual difficulties. *The Journal of Sex Research, 55*(6), 783–801. https://doi.org/10.1080/00224499.2017.1410519

Medina-Perucha, L., Yousaf, O., Hunter, M., & Grunfeld, E. (2017). Barriers to medical help-seeking among older men with prostate cancer. *Journal of Psychosocial Oncology, 35*(5), 531–543. https://doi.org/10.1080/07347332.2017.1312661

Men's Pie Club. (2024). *Men's Pie Club.* https://www.menspieclub.co.uk/about

Men's Sheds. (2024). *Men's Sheds.* https://menssheds.org.uk/

Mental Health Foundation. (2023). *Millions of men in the UK affected by body image issues—Mental Health Foundation survey.* https://www.mentalhealth.org.uk/about-us/news/millions-men-uk-affected-body-image-issues-mental-health-foundation-survey

Mergl, R., Koburger, N., Heinrichs, K., Székely, A., Tóth, M. D., Coyne, J., Quintão, S., Arensman, E., Coffey, C., Maxwell, M., Värnik, A., Van Audenhove, C., McDaid, D., Sarchiapone, M., Schmidtke, A., Genz, A., Gusmão, R., & Hegerl, U. (2015). What are reasons for the large gender differences in the lethality of suicidal acts? An epidemiological analysis in four European countries. *PLoS ONE, 10*(7). https://doi.org/10.1371/JOURNAL.PONE.0129062

Milligan, C., Neary, D., Payne, S., Hanratty, B., Irwin, P., & Dowrick, C. (2016). Older men and social activity: A scoping review of Men's Sheds and other gendered interventions. *Ageing and Society, 36*(5), 895–923. https://doi.org/10.1017/S0144686X14001524

Minns Lowe, C. J., Toye, F., & Barker, K. L. (2019). Men's experiences of having osteoporosis vertebral fractures: A qualitative study using interpretative phenomenological analyses. *Osteoporosis International, 30*(7), 1403–1412. https://doi.org/10.1007/S00198-019-04973-0

Mitchell, G., Ferguson-Pare, M., & Richards, J. (2003). Exploring an alternative metaphor for nursing: Relinquishing military images and language. *Nursing Leadership (Toronto, Ont.), 16*(1), 48–58.

Modell, A. H. (2005). Emotional memory, metaphor, and meaning. *Psychoanalytic Inquiry, 25*(4), 555–568.

Moisio, R., Arnould, E., & Gentry, J. (2013). Productive consumption in the class-mediated construction of domestic masculinity: Do-it-yourself (DIY) home improvement in men's identity work. *Journal of Consumer Research, 40*(2), 298–316.

Molzahn, A. E., Starzomski, R., McDonald, M., & O'Loughlin, C. (2005). Chinese Canadian beliefs toward organ donation. *Qualitative Health Research, 15*(1), 82–98.

Newman, C. E., Gray, R., Brener, L., Jackson, L. C., Dillon, A., Saunders, V., Johnson, P., & Treloar, C. (2017). "I had a little bit of a bloke meltdown…But the next day, i was up": Understanding cancer experiences among aboriginal men. *Cancer Nursing, 40*(3), E1–E8. https://doi.org/10.1097/NCC.0000000000000399

NIHR. (2022, January). *Improving inclusion of under-served groups in clinical research: Guidance from INCLUDE project.* https://www.NIHR.ac.UK/documents/improving-Inclusion-of-under-served-groups-in-clinical-research-guidance-from-include-project/25435.

O'Brien, R., Hart, G. J., & Hunt, K. (2007). "Standing out from the herd": Men renegotiating masculinity in relation to their experience of illness. *International Journal of Men's Health, 6*(3), 178–200.

O'Brien, R., Hunt, K., & Hart, G. (2005). 'It's caveman stuff, but that is to a certain extent how guys still operate': Men's accounts of masculinity and help seeking. *Social Science & Medicine, 61*(3), 503–516.

OECD. (2017). *Health at a glance 2017: OECD indicators.*

Oliffe, J. (2005). Constructions of masculinity following prostatectomy-induced impotence. *Social Science & Medicine, 60*(10), 2249–2259. https://doi.org/10.1016/J.SOCSCIMED.2004.10.016

Oliffe, J. (2006). Embodied masculinity and androgen deprivation therapy. *Sociology of Health & Illness, 28*(4), 410–432. https://doi.org/10.1111/J.1467-9566.2006.00499.X

Oliffe, J., & Mróz, L. (2005). Men interviewing men about health and illness: Ten lessons learned. *The Journal of Men's Health & Gender, 2*(2), 257–260.

Oliffe, J., Rossnagel, E., Bottorff, J., Chambers, S., Caperchione, C., & Rice, S. (2020). Community-based men's health promotion programs: Eight lessons learnt and their caveats. *Health Promotion International, 35*, 1230–1240.

Oliffe, J. L., Ogrodniczuk, J., Bottorff, J. L., Hislop, T. G., & Halpin, M. (2009). Connecting humor, health, and masculinities at prostate cancer support groups. *Psycho-Oncology, 18*(9), 916–926. https://doi.org/10.1002/pon.1415

Oliffe, J. L., Rasmussen, B., Bottorff, J. L., Kelly, M. T., Galdas, P. M., Phinney, A., & Ogrodniczuk, J. S. (2013). Masculinities, work, and retirement among older men who experience depression. *Qualitative Health Research, 23*(12), 1626–1637. https://doi.org/10.1177/1049732313509408

Östlund, G., Björk, M., Valtersson, E., & Sverker, A. (2015). Lived experiences of sex life difficulties in men and women with early RA—The Swedish TIRA project. *Musculoskeletal Care, 13*(4), 248–257. https://doi.org/10.1002/MSC.1105

Otto, M. W. (2000). Stories and metaphors in cognitive-behavior therapy. *Cognitive and Behavioral Practice, 7*(2), 166–172.

Paulson, M., Norberg, A., & Danielson, E. (2002). Men living with fibromyalgia-type pain: Experiences as patients in the Swedish health care system. *Journal of Advanced Nursing, 40*(1), 87–95. https://doi.org/10.1046/j.1365-2648.2002.02343.x

Perez-Garcia, F. L., Röder, E., Pastoor, H., Bolt, J. M., van Exel, J., & Dolhain, E. M. R. J. (2021). It is not just about sex: Viewpoints of men with inflammatory arthritis on the overall impact of the disease on their sexual health Inflammatory arthritis. *RMD Open, 7*. https://doi.org/10.1136/rmdopen-2021-001821

Peterson, J. W., & Sterling, Y. M. (2009). Children's perceptions of asthma: African American children use metaphors to make sense of asthma. *Journal of Pediatric Health Care, 23*(2), 93–100.

Piemonte, N. M. (2015). Last laughs: Gallows humor and medical education. *Journal of Medical Humanities, 36*(4), 375–390. https://doi.org/10.1007/S10912-015-9338-4

Pierz, A. J., Randall, T. C., Castle, P. E., Adedimeji, A., Ingabire, C., Kubwimana, G., Uwinkindi, F., Hagenimana, M., Businge, L., Musabyimana, F., Munyaneza, A., & Murenzi, G. (2020). A scoping review: Facilitators and barriers of cervical cancer screening and early diagnosis of breast cancer in Sub-Saharan African health settings. *Gynecologic Oncology Reports, 33*, 100605. https://doi.org/10.1016/J.GORE.2020.100605

Pollack, W. S. (1998). *Real boys: Rescuing our sons from the myths of boyhood*. Henry Holt and Company.

Potter, A. M., Bentz, B., Crue, L., Leiby, S., Bashi, S., Maguire, K., Meyers, J., & Mieczkowski, K. (2023). Men's lived experiences of breast cancer and changes in occupation. *Occupational Therapy International*. https://doi.org/10.1155/2023/9641922

Primholdt, N., Primdahl, J., & Hendricks, O. (2017). A difficult diagnosis: A qualitative study of the daily lives of young men diagnosed with ankylosing spondylitis. *Musculoskeletal Care, 15*(2), 140–149. https://doi.org/10.1002/MSC.1155

Prior, J. A., Crawford-Manning, F., Whittle, R., Abdul-Sultan, A., Chew-Graham, C. A., Muller, S., Shepherd, T. A., Sumathipala, A., Mallen, C. D., & Paskins, Z. (2021). Vertebral fracture as a risk factor for self-harm: A retrospective cohort study. *BMC Musculoskeletal Disorders, 22*(1). https://doi.org/10.1186/S12891-021-04631-9

Quaglia, V. (2020). Men, masculinities and diabetes: 'Doing gender' in Italian men's narratives of chronic illness. *Sociology of Health & Illness, 42*(8), 1902–1917. https://doi.org/10.1111/1467-9566.13176

Quincey, K., Williamson, I., & Wildbur, D. (2021). Men with breast cancer and their encounters with masculinity: An interpretative phenomenological analysis using photography. *Psychology of Men and Masculinity, 22*(4), 690–703. https://doi.org/10.1037/MEN0000344

Quincey, K., Williamson, I., & Winstanley, S. (2016). 'Marginalised malignancies': A qualitative synthesis of men's accounts of living with breast cancer. *Social Science & Medicine, 149*, 17–25. https://doi.org/10.1016/J.SOCSCIMED.2015.11.032

Randles, J. (2018). "Manning up" to be a good father: Hybrid fatherhood, masculinity, and U.S. responsible fatherhood policy. *Gender and Society, 32*(4), 516–539. https://doi.org/10.1177/0891243218770364

Rao, D., Feinglass, J., & Corrigan, P. (2007). Racial and ethnic disparities in mental illness stigma. *Journal of Nervous and Mental Disease, 195*(12), 1020–1023. https://doi.org/10.1097/NMD.0b013e31815c046e

Reisfield, G. M., & Wilson, G. R. (2004). Use of metaphor in the discourse on cancer. *Journal of Clinical Oncology, 22*(19), 4024–4027.

Rennie, C., Stoddart, K., & Hubbard, G. (2018). A new normal: Reconciling change in appearance and function for men with head and neck cancer. *Cancer Nursing Practice, 17*(5). https://doi.org/10.7748/cnp.2018.e1449

Richards, H., & Emslie, C. (2000). The 'doctor' or the 'girl from the university'? Considering the influence of professional roles on qualitative interviewing. *Family Practice, 17*(1), 71–75.

Richardson, J., & Grose, J. (2009). The use of descriptive words and metaphor in patient and carer experience of palliative day care: Secondary analysis of a qualitative study. *The Open Nursing Journal, 3*, 18–24.

Ridge, D., Emslie, C., & White, A. (2011). Understanding how men experience, express and cope with mental distress: Where next? *Sociology of Health & Illness, 33*(1), 145–159.

Rivas, C., Matheson, L., Nayoan, J., Glaser, A., Gavin, A., Wright, P., Wagland, R., & Watson, E. (2016). Ethnicity and the prostate cancer experience: A qualitative metasynthesis. In *Psycho-Oncology* (Vol. 25, Issue 10, pp. 1147–1156). https://doi.org/10.1002/pon.4222

Robertson, C., Archibald, D., Avenell, A., Douglas, F., Hoddinott, P., Boyers, D., Stewart, F., Boachie, C., Fioratou, E., & Wilkins, D. (2014). Systematic reviews of and integrated report on the quantitative, qualitative and economic evidence base for the management of obesity in men. *Health Technology Assessment, 18*(35), 1–458.

Robertson, S. (2007). *Understanding men and health: Masculinities, identity and well-being*. Open University Press.

Robertson, S., Sheikh, K., & Moore, A. (2010). Embodied masculinities in the context of cardiac rehabilitation. *Sociology of Health & Illness, 32*(5), 695–710. https://doi.org/10.1111/j.1467-9566.2010.01249.x

Rochlen, A., Paterniti, D., Epstein, R., Duberstein, P., Willeford, L., & Kravitz, R. (2010). Barriers in diagnosing and treating men with depression: A focus group report. *American Journal of Men's Health, 4*(2), 167–175. https://doi.org/10.1177/1557988309335823

Salifu, Y., Almack, K., & Caswell, G. (2023). 'Out of the frying pan into the fire': A qualitative study of the impact on masculinity for men living with advanced prostate cancer. *Palliative Care and Social Practice, 17.* https://doi.org/10.1177/26323524231176829/

Sallinen, M., Mengshoel, A. M., & Solbrække, K. N. (2019). "I can't have it; I am a man. A young man!"—men, fibromyalgia and masculinity in a Nordic context. *International Journal of Qualitative Studies on Health and Well-Being, 14*(1). https://doi.org/10.1080/17482631.2019.1676974

Sattar, S., Haase, K., Bradley, C., Papadopoulos, E., Kuster, S., Mina, D., Tippe, M., Kaur, A., Campbell, D., Joshua, A., Rediger, C., Souied, O., & Alibhai, S. (2023). Barriers and facilitators related to undertaking physical activities among men with prostate cancer: A scoping review. *Prostate Cancer and Prostatic Diseases, 24*, 1007–1027.

Schrock, D., & Schwalbe, M. (2009). Men, masculinity, and manhood acts. *Annual Review of Sociology, 35*, 277–295.

Schwalbe, M., & Wolkomir, M. (2001). The masculine self as problem and resource in interview studies of men. *Men and Masculinities, 4*(1), 90–103.

Seale, C. (2006). Gender accommodation in online cancer support groups. *Health, 10*(3), 345–360. https://doi.org/10.1177/1363459306064495

Sharf, B., Stelljes, L., & Gordon, H. (2005). "A little bitty spot and I'm a big man": Patients' perspectives on refusing diagnosis or treatment for lung cancer. *Psycho-Oncology, 14*(8), 636–646. https://doi.org/10.1002/pon.885

Sharp, P., Bottorff, J. L., Rice, S., Oliffe, J. L., Schulenkorf, N., Impellizzeri, F., & Caperchione, C. M. (2022). "People say men don't talk, well that's bullshit": A focus group study exploring challenges and opportunities for men's mental health promotion. *PLOS ONE, 17*(1), e0261997. https://doi.org/10.1371/JOURNAL.PONE.0261997

Sigurdsson, B., Palsson, S. P., Aevarsson, O., Olafsdottir, M., & Johannsson, M. (2015). Validity of Gotland Male Depression Scale for male depression in a community study: The Sudurnesjamenn study. *Journal of Affective Disorders, 173*, 81–89.

Snell, G. E., Seage, C. H., & Mercer, J. (2023). A phenomenological study on the lived experience of men with chronic fatigue syndrome. *Journal of Health Psychology.* https://doi.org/10.1177/13591053231186385

Staiger, T., Stiawa, M., Mueller-Stierlin, A. S., Kilian, R., Beschoner, P., Gündel, H., Becker, T., Frasch, K., Panzirsch, M., Schmauß, M., & Krumm, S. (2020). Masculinity and help-seeking among men with depression: A qualitative study. *Frontiers in Psychiatry, 11.* https://doi.org/10.3389/FPSYT.2020.599039

Stand up to cancer. (2023). *Stand up to cancer.* https://www.standuptocancer.org.uk/

Stapleton, S., & Pattison, N. (2014). The lived experience of men with advanced cancer in relation to their perceptions of masculinity: A qualitative phenomenological study. *Journal of Clinical Nursing, 24*(7–8), 1069–1078. https://doi.org/10.1111/jocn.12713

Talk Club. (2024). *Talk Club*. https://talkclub.org/

Tang, M., Oliffe, J., Galdas, P., Phinney, A., & Han, C. (2014). College men's depression-related help-seeking: A gender analysis. *Journal of Mental Health, 23*(5), 219–224. https://doi.org/10.3109/09638237.2014.910639

Tang, P. L., Wang, H. H., & Chou, F. H. (2015). A Systematic review and meta-analysis of demoralization and depression in patients with cancer. *Psychosomatics, 56*(6), 634–643. https://doi.org/10.1016/J.PSYM.2015.06.005

Tarrant, A. (2013). Grandfathering as spatio-temporal practice: Conceptualizing performances of ageing masculinities in contemporary familial carescapes. *Social & Cultural Geography, 14*(2), 192–210.

Thomeer, M. B., Reczek, C., & Umberson, D. (2015). Relationship dynamics around depression in gay and lesbian couples. *Social Science and Medicine, 147*, 38–46. https://doi.org/10.1016/j.socscimed.2015.10.048

Thongtang, P., Fongkaew, W., Sansiriphun, N., & Chaloumsuk, N. (2021). My thing is dead: Experience of dealing with diabetic erectile dysfunction of northern Thai men. *Pacific Rim International Journal of Nursing Research, 25*(2), 255–268.

Törnävä, M., Harju, E., Vasarainen, H., Pakarainen, T., Perttilä, I., & Kaipia, A. (2022). Men's experiences of the impact of penile cancer surgery on their lives: A qualitative study. *European Journal of Cancer Care, 31*(1), e13548. https://doi.org/10.1111/ECC.13548

Toye, F., Room, J., & Barker, K. L. (2017). Do I really want to be going on a bloody diet? Gendered narratives in older men with painful knee osteoarthritis. *Disability and Rehabilitation, 40*(16), 1914–1920. https://doi.org/10.1080/09638288.2017.1323017

Trusson, D., & Quincey, K. (2021). Breast cancer and hair loss: Experiential similarities and differences in men's and women's narratives. *Cancer Nursing, 44*(1), 62–70.

Vigorito, A. J., & Curry, T. J. (1998). Marketing masculinity: Gender identity and popular magazines. *Sex Roles, 39*(1–2), 135–152.

Wagland, R., Nayoan, J., Matheson, L., Rivas, C., Brett, J., Collaco, N., Alexis, O., Gavin, A., Glaser, A. W., & Watson, E. (2019). Adjustment strategies amongst black African and black Caribbean men following treatment for prostate cancer: Findings from the Life After Prostate Cancer Diagnosis. *European Journal of Cancer Care, 29*(1). https://doi.org/10.1111/ecc.13183

Wagner, P. (2016). Picture perfect bodies: Visualizing hegemonic masculinities produced for/by male fitness spaces. *International Journal of Men's Health, 15*(3), 235–258.

Walker, A. Q., Blake, C. E., Moore, J. B., Wilcox, S., DuBois, K., Watkins, W., & K. (2022). Experiences of midlife and older African American men living with type 2 diabetes. *Ethnicity & Health, 27*(6), 1256–1270. https://doi.org/10.1080/13557858.2021.1910206

Wang, Y., Freemantle, N., Nazareth, I., & Hunt, K. (2014). Gender differences in survival and the use of primary care prior to diagnosis of three cancers: An analysis of routinely collected UK general practice data. *PLOS ONE, 9*(7), e101562.

Warner, L. R., & Shields, S. A. (2007). The perception of crying in women and men: Angry tears, sad tears, and the "right way" to cry. In U. Hess & P. Philippot (Eds.), *Group dynamics and emotional expression* (pp. 92–117). Cambridge University Press.

Watson, K. (2011). Gallows humor in medicine. *Hastings Center Report, 41*(5), 37–45.

Watts, S., & Stenner, P. (2012). *Doing Q methodological research: Theory, method and interpretation*. Sage.

Wenger, L. (2013). "Living under assault": Men making sense of cancer. *European Journal of Cancer Care, 22*, 389–399. https://doi.org/10.1111/ecc.12042

Wenger, L., & Oliffe, J. (2013). Men managing cancer: A gender analysis. *Sociology of Health & Illness, 36*(1), 108–122. https://doi.org/10.1111/1467-9566.12045

Wennick, A., Jönsson, A. K., Bratt, O., & Stenzelius, K. (2017). Everyday life after a radical prostatectomy—A qualitative study of men under 65 years of age. *European Journal of Oncology Nursing, 30*, 107–112. https://doi.org/10.1016/J.EJON.2017.08.008

Whaley, B. B. (2000). Explaining illness to children: Theory, strategies, and future inquiry. In B. B. Whaley (Ed.), *Explaining illness: Research, theory and strategies* (Vol. Issue 2, pp. 191–203). Lawrence Erlbaum Associates.

White, A. (2007). Men and the problems of late diagnosis. In J. Heidelbaugh (Ed.), *Clinical men's health: Evidence in practice* (1st ed., pp. 31–43). Elsevier.

White, A., & Banks, I. (2009). Men and help seeking. In R. Kirby, C. Carson III, A. White, & M. Kirby (Eds.), *Men's health* (3rd ed., pp. 505–514). CRC Press.

White, A., De Sousa, B., De Visser, R., Hogston, R., Madsen, S. A., Makara, P., McKee, M., Raine, G., Richardson, N., & Clarke, N. (2011). Men's health in Europe. *Journal of Men's Health, 8*(3), 192–201.

White, A. K., & Johnson, M. (2000). Men making sense of their chest pain—niggles, doubts and denials. *Journal of Clinical Nursing, 9*(4), 534–541. https://doi.org/10.1046/j.1365-2702.2000.00413.x

Wills, T. A. (1981). Downward comparison principles in social psychology. *Psychological Bulletin, 90*(2), 245–271.

Wills, T. A. (1987). Downward comparison as a coping mechanism. In C. R. Snyder & C. Ford (Eds.), *Coping with negative life events: Clinical and social-psychological perspectives*. Plenum Press.

Wilson, O., Kirwan, J., Dures, E., Quest, E., & Hewlett, S. (2017). The experience of foot problems and decisions to access foot care in patients with rheumatoid arthritis: A qualitative study. *Journal of Foot and Ankle Research, 10*(1), 1–11. https://doi.org/10.1186/S13047-017-0188-3

Witty, K., Branney, P., Bullen, K., White, A., Evans, J., & Eardley, I. (2014). Engaging men with penile cancer in qualitative research: Reflections from an interview-based study. *Nurse Researcher, 21*(3), 13–19.

Wong, Y. J., & Rochlen, A. B. (2005). Demystifying men's emotional behavior: New directions and implications for counseling and research. *Psychology of Men & Masculinity, 6*, 62–72.

World Health Organisation. (2023a). *Nurses by sex (%)*. https://www.WHO.int/data/GHO/data/indicators/indicator-details/GHO/nurses-by-sex-(-)

World Health Organisation. (2023b). *Sexual and reproductive health and research*. https://www.WHO.int/teams/sexual-and-reproductive-health-and-research/key-areas-of-work/sexual-health/defining-sexual-health

Wurmser, L. (2011). Metaphor as conflict, conflict as metaphor. *Psychoanalytic Inquiry, 31*(2), 107–125. https://doi.org/10.1080/07351690.2010.515528

Yaklin, S., Kim, M., & Social, J. H. (2022). African American men who become mental health advocates. *International Journal of Social Psychiatry, 68*(5), 981–990. https://doi.org/10.1177/00207640211012736

Yelland, C., & Tiggemann, M. (2003). Muscularity and the gay ideal: Body dissatisfaction and disordered eating in homosexual men. *Eating Behaviors, 4*(2), 107–116. https://doi.org/10.1016/S1471-0153(03)00014-X

Yip, K., & Navarro-Millán, I. (2021). Racial, ethnic, and healthcare disparities in rheumatoid arthritis. *Current Opinion in Rheumatology, 33*(2), 117–121. https://doi.org/10.1097/BOR.0000000000000782

Young, M. D., Morgan, P. J., Plotnikoff, R. C., Callister, R., & Collins, C. E. (2012). Effectiveness of male-only weight loss and weight loss maintenance interventions: A systematic review with meta-analysis. *Obesity Reviews, 13*(5), 393–408.

Yousaf, O., Grunfeld, E., & Hunter, M. (2013). A systematic review of the factors associated with delays in medical and psychological help-seeking among men. *Health Psychology Review, 9*(2), 264–276. https://doi.org/10.1080/17437199.2013.840954

Zierau, F., Bille, A., Rutz, W., & Bech, P. (2002). The Gotland male depression scale: A validity study in patients with alcohol use disorder. *Nordic Journal of Psychiatry, 56*(4), 265–271.

Zucchelli, F., Sharratt, N., Montgomery, K., & Chambers, J. (2022). Men's experiences of alopecia areata: A qualitative study. *Health Psychology Open, 1–13*. https://doi.org/10.1177/20551029221121524

Index

C. Flurey, *Talking Men's Health*,
https://doi.org/10.1007/978-3-031-62593-0

The manufacturer's authorised representative in the EU is Springer Nature Customer Service Centre GmbH, Europaplatz 3, 69115 Heidelberg, Germany. If you have any concerns regarding our products, please contact ProductSafety@springernature.com

Printed and bound by CPI Group (UK) Ltd, Croydon, CR0 4YY
01/10/2026
02225903-0007